Hospital Management and Administration

ABOUT THE AUTHOR

Santosh Lyall did M.Com, and obtained MBA in Hospitality from IITM. After practicing as independent educator and consultant, he joined as director at Ideal Institute of Management, Ghazibad. Presently he is Director of Sardar Bhagat Singh Institute of Management and Technology, Noida. He has ample experience of running executive programmes for many corporate houses on Organization Behaviour, Stretegic Management, Organization, Planning and Material Management. He has authored many books on various topics of management. His articles are well praised as and when they appears in newspapers and magazines.

ABOUT THE BOOK

Hospital management and administration is concerned with the organization, coordination, planning, staffing, evaluating and controlling of health services for the masses. The primary objective is to provide quality healthcare to people and that too in a cost-effective manner. Professional hospital administrators have proven how institutions can be managed proficiently, economically and successfully in a given time period. Hospital represents any institution duly licensed, certified and operated as a hospital. Hospital case management is a collaborative process that assesses, plans, implements, coordinates, monitors and evaluates the options and services required to meet an individual's health needs using communication and available resources to promote quality, cost-effective outcomes in the hospital environment. Hospital care is a service provided by a coordinated group of doctors, paramedical staff, nurses, technicians, supportive and administrative workers to the people suffering from physical, mental and social ailments. The level of care depends on the skill and clinical acumen of the physician and his team as well as equipment and infrastructure facilities. This book targets those in healthcare professions and health services management, providing them with a reliable handbook on efficient managerial practices.

Hospital Management and Administration

Santosh Lyall

AMIGA PRESS INC.
Delhi-110051

AMIGA PRESS INC.
Regd. Office: - 28-A, Indra Park, St.No-9
Near-Chander Nagar, Krishna Nagar
Delhi : - 110051 (India)
Tel : - 011-22040120, 22504028, +91-98736-57000
Email : - amigapress@gmail.com
info@amigapress.co.in
amigaeditorial@gmail.com
amigapub@gmail.com
Website : - www.amigapress.co.in

Sales and Marketing Office : - 89 Gyan Park, Chander Nagar
Krishna Nagar, Delhi- 110051

This edition is published by Amiga Press Inc.

ISBN: 978-93-87295-66-7

First Published 2020

Printed and bound by Amiga Press Inc.

Preface

Hospital represents any institution duly licensed, certified and operated as a hospital. Hospital case management is a collaborative process that assesses, plans, implements, coordinates, monitors and evaluates the options and services required to meet an individual's health needs using communication and available resources to promote quality, cost-effective outcomes in the hospital environment.

Management of such a complex organization requires blending of technical and administrative competence in the right quantity, at the right time, at the right place, by the right men and in the right way or process. Each hospital is a distinct entity and as such each has to be tailored to the specific aims to be accomplished, the specific tasks to be performed, the volume of services to be rendered and the type of community to be served.

Moreover, there is manifold increase in the complexity and processes that take place in the successful management of a modern day hospital. This in turn has lead to a tremendous demand for efficient professionals who can handle the day-to-day chores of hospital management and administration. Highly trained professionals are needed for the smooth operating of a hospital.

Hospital doors are always open. No matter what time of day, hospital physicians and staff need to be prepared for anything – from treating life-threatening diseases or the common cold, to aiding in emergency situations and disaster relief. With several departments all providing life-saving care, operating complex equipment, and handling business issues like policy development and compliance, hospitals need top-notch management to help them run efficiently. That's why a position in Hospital Management is so important, not only for the patients, but also for medical professionals and the healthcare system as a whole.

Usually, those starting their studies with sights set on a position in hospital management choose to pursue a Bachelor of Science in Healthcare

Administration for a solid base and foundation in medical and business studies. On the undergraduate level, courses cover topics around managed care, community health, medical research, accounting, healthcare finance, medical marketing, and planning. At this level, students should be focusing their studies both inside and outside the classroom, looking to secure quality internship or fellowship experiences within the type of hospital setting where they would like to work.

Health administration, healthcare administration, healthcare management or hospital management is the field relating to leadership, management, and administration of public health systems, health care systems, hospitals,and hospital networks in all the primary, secondary, and tertiary sectors.

Health systems management ensures that specific outcomes are attained, that departments within a health facility are running smoothly, that the right people are in the right jobs, that people know what is expected of them, that resources are used efficiently and that all departments are working towards a common goal for mutual development and growth.

A Hospital administrator is overall in charge of administrative affairs of the hospital. He takes over the charge of various aspects of health administration and hospital administration with respect to patients and healthcare.

This is a reference book. All the matter is just compiled and edited in nature, taken from the various sources which are in public domain.

This book targets those in healthcare professions and health services management, providing them with a reliable handbook on efficient managerial practices.

—Editor

Contents

1

Introduction

FUNCTIONS OF THE HOSPITAL

To Provide Care for the Sick and Injured

This can be done by accommodating them according to their physical condition and financial status. When we talk of physical condition, we mean that some patients are seriously ill and require admission in Intensive Care Unit while others are not so seriously ill and can be' accommodated elsewhere (*e.g.* in deluxe room, single room with AC and without AC, semi-private room and general ward) according to their financial status. There may be some patients who may require isolation. In that case, they should be kept in isolated rooms, but the building should be kept always in a good state of repair, pleasing appearance and providing the patient every mental and physical comfort.

In every hospital, there should be sufficient diagnostic and treatment facilities available such as medical laboratory, X-ray, ultrasound, MRI and CT scan for diagnosis, and operation theatre for surgery, labour room for delivery, nursery for children, physical therapy for rehabilitation of patients, so that they may be properly treated.

Training of Physicians, Nurses and other Personnel

They receive their training in both theory and practice in approved schools and colleges. Therefore, a hospital being a complex and specialized organization must employ highly trained personnel so that they may train others. Particularly in the branch of medical and paramedical education, different associations/councils play very important roles.

They make surveys of hospitals and accord their approval. Only these approved hospitals can provide training in medicine, nursing, dietetics, pharmacy, physiotherapy, administration, medical social work, medical record library, X-ray and medical record technology, etc. Capable boys and girls should be attracted to such courses as a career which offers them fair remuneration, opportunities for self-development and reasonable security.

Prevention of Disease and Promotion of Health

It is the duty of the hospital to cooperate with the government agencies. They can treat patients of communicable and non-communicable diseases, notify to the recognized authorities of any communicable disease of which it has knowledge, assist in vaccination programmes of the government, etc.

Advancement of Research in Scientific Medicine

In light of the broad social responsibility for maintaining and restoring the health, it is an important function, but no hospital is permitted to do direct experiments on patients. It must resort to necessary tests in laboratories and on animals. They can do so by making observations of functions of the body in health and in disease but they will have to main clinical record of patients accurately for which they have to engage qualified trained medical record technicians who will preserve the record in such a manner that it can be made available for study at any time to physicians and surgeons.

COMPLICATIONS IN HOSPITAL FUNCTION

A hospital has many organizational and operational elements in common with hotels, industrial organizations and educational institutions. However, a hospital is a unique institution as it includes all activities present in each of the groups.

The difference between administrative work in hospitals and in other organizations can be attributed to the existence of the following conditions peculiar to hospitals:

- The consumers of the services provided in a hospital (the patients) are physically or mentally ill and are rendered services within the four walls of the hospital. As compared with most other institutions of business, government and education, this is an unusual situation and presents quite different problems of management.
- The customers of the hospital (the patients) have individual needs and require highly personalized and custom-made services, the

diagnostic, therapeutic and preventive services provided by physicians, nurses and technicians, with the aid of expensive and specialized equipments and medication are needs of each individual consumer.

- In addition to the more common institutional services and functions such as food preparation, general housekeeping, laundry, maintenance, purchasing, personnel, credit and collection and public relations, the hospital also provides a wide range of scientific and technical services such as nursing, diet therapy, anesthesiology, pharmacy, radiology, clinical laboratory, physiotherapy and medical social work. Also, many of its services are provided continuously, round the clock, every day of the year.
- All these services involve many individuals-the ill customer himself, his emotionally tense relatives and friends, physicians, technologists, clerks and manual labourers. These individuals are working, suffering, eating and sleeping within a comparatively small space and in an unusual atmosphere, highly charged with emotion and tension. Only a very capable administrator can adequately understand and effectively deal with the human relations problems arising from these constraints.
- Nurses and certain other personnel must accept direction from both the matron and the physicians under whom they work closely every day. The human relations problems in such situations of dual authority are much more frequent, delicate, varied and complex than in organizations where this situation does not exist.
- Handicapped by low wages, rigid discipline and some apprehension of exposure to disease, hospital personnel are expected to maintain a very high level of efficiency, as their functioning affects the lives of patients.
- Another way in which the responsibilities and activities of the hospital administrator differ from his counterpart in other fields is in the amount and variety of training programmes that the hospital has to provide. Training is provided for medical interns and residents (6 months to 1 year), nurses (3 to 4 years), X-ray technicians (2 years), medical laboratory technicians (2 years), physiotherapists (4 years), pharmacists (2 years), medical social workers (2 years), dieticians (2 years), nurse aides and nursing orderlies (1 year). Classroom, clinical and apprenticeship training methods are used in varying combinations. The administrator is

responsible for planning and operating these various training programmes. Very few other types of institutions combine such major educational responsibilities with other operating activities.

- Just as administration in hospitals differs from that in most other fields, similarly, public relations aspects and problems of hospitals are more pervasive, delicate and volatile. The human elements- the consumers (patients), producers of care and services (doctors, nurses and other personnel), the variety of community health agencies, the other competing hospitals, the people in the community (relatives and friends of the patients)- and the conditions and environment in which they are brought together (the hospital), present public relations problems of a sort and variety vastly different from those of most other institutions.
- The efficiency and quality of health care services in any hospital is directly dependent on the use of bio-medical equipments in diagnosis, surgery and therapeutic process. These equipments invariably employ sophisticated technology made of complex systems. Hence, the problem of maintenance and management of these bio-medical equipments is complex because there is acute shortage of technical hands who have suitable and adequate training in the maintenance and repairing of these specialized hi-tech equipments. At times, spare parts and components are not available because the models of these equipments undergo frequent change. Next, the local dealers in India by and large do not provide worthwhile after sales service or repair. The poor hospital administrator is in a fix whether to go for hi-tech bio-medical equipments or use conventional methods of treatment. If he opts for the first, he either discards these equipments one after another in view of the factors, or enhances the cost of treatment. If he does not opt for hi-tech biomedical equipments, he loses his clientele.
- The introduction of Consumer Protection Act, 1986 and subsequently, the Supreme Court judgement bringing doctors under the purview of this act have evoked diverse reactions. While the public is happy about what they call it a long overdue judgement; but the doctors and hospital administrators are not happy at all as it will worsen the patientdoctor relationship and surely increase the cost of treatment. The poor hospital administrator will have to attend consumer courts for no rhyme or reason in most of the cases as the patients are not only misled by advocates, but the

consumer courts issue notices to doctors and hospitals without understanding the nature of complaints filed by patients. In other institutions, such as hotel or industry chief executives can explain to the advocate, in their office, the line of defence to be taken in the consumer courts before the trial begins, but in case of hospitals, their hospital administrators will have to stand by the side of their advocates to explain each step taken in the treatment of patients by doctors, as neither the advocates nor the judges of the consumer courts possess any medical expertise.

- Hospital waste management is another peculiar condition to administrative work in hospital and has become a burning issue these days for hospital administrators, as increased awareness of health and its related problems amongst the general public has led to the demand for comprehensive health care facilities which in turn require frequent visits to hospitals by the patients to undergo various tests. This results in the escalating amount of hospital waste generation in the environment. This hospital waste is not like domestic waste, but a potentially hazardous waste. Its unscientific disposal can pose serious problems to the public in general, and the hospital administrator in particular, as it results in increased morbidity due to chemical and radioactive toxicity in the environment and transmission of various diseases. The conventional waste disposal method does not work at all. Hence the hospital administrator faces another peculiar problem what is not faced by a chief executive of a business organization or a hotel in disposing of the waste of their institutions.

This distinctiveness of hospital administrations, call for a high degree of professional competence to do justice to the job. It is, therefore, obvious that hospital administration should be entrusted to those who have the necessary training and the right kind of attitude to perform this vital task.

CLASSIFICATION OF HOSPITALS

Hospitals have been classified in many ways.

The most commonly accepted criteria for the classification of the modern hospitals are:

- Length of stay of patients (long-term or short-term),
- Clinical basis, and

- Ownership control basis. The following is a discussion on the third aspect.

Classification According to Ownership/Control

On the basis of ownership or control, hospitals can be divided into four categories, namely, public hospitals, voluntary hospitals, private nursing homes and corporate hospitals.

Public Hospitals

Public hospitals are those run by the Central Government, state governments or local bodies on non-commercial lines. These hospitals may be general hospitals or specialized hospitals or both. General hospitals are those which provide treatment for common diseases, whereas specialized hospitals provide treatment for specific diseases like infectious diseases, cancer, eye diseases, psychiatric ailments, etc. General hospitals can diagnose patients suffering from infectious diseases, but refer them to infectious disease hospitals for hospitalization, as general hospitals are not licensed to treat infectious-diseased patients.

Voluntary Hospitals

Voluntary hospitals are those which are established and incorporated under the Societies Registration Act, 1860 or Public Trust Act, 1882 or any other appropriate Act of the Central or state government. They are run with public or private funds on a non-commercial basis. No part of the profit of the voluntary hospital goes to the benefit of any member, trustee or to any other individual. Similarly, no member, trustee or any other individual is entitled to a share in the distribution of any of the, corporate assets on dissolution of the registered society.

A board of trustees, usually comprising prominent members of the community and retired high officials of the government, manages such hospitals. The board appoints an administrator and a medical director to run such voluntary hospitals. These hospitals spend more on patient care than what they receive from the patients.

There is, of late, a trend among voluntary hospitals to charge reasonably high fees from rich patients and very little from poor patients. Whatever they earn from the rich patients of the private wards, spend on the patients of general wards. However, the main sources of their revenue are public and private donations, and grants-in-aid from the Central Government, the state government, and from philanthropic organizations, both national and international. Thus, voluntary hospitals run on a 'no profit, no loss' basis.

Private Nursing Homes

Private nursing homes are generally owned by an individual doctor or a group of doctors. They admit patients suffering from infirmity, advanced age, illness, injury, chronic disability, etc., or those who are convalescing, but they do not admit patients suffering from communicable diseases, alcoholism, drug-addiction or mental illness. There is, however, no uniform definition for nursing homes.

The phrase may refer to out-of-home care facilities that offer a range of services similar to many found in a hospital. These nursing homes are run on a commercial basis. Naturally, the ordinary citizen cannot usually afford to get medical treatment there. However, these nursing homes are becoming more and more popular due to the shortage of government and voluntary hospitals. Secondly, wealthy patients do not want to get treatment at public hospitals due to long queues of patients and the shortage of medical as well as nursing staff leading to lack of medical and nursing care.

Corporate Hospitals

The latest concept is of corporate hospitals which are public limited companies formed under the Companies Act. They are normally run on commercial lines.

They can be either general or specialized or both:

- What is Trust Hospital?
- Where the Hospital is registered under The Bombay Public Trusts Act, 1950, it is considered to be Trust Hospital.

The Bombay Public Trusts Act, 1950 provides machinery of charity commissioners to regulate the administration of public religious and charitable trusts. It makes registration of all the public religious and charitable trusts including the religious trusts created under Hindu Muslim and Christian personal laws mandatory and prescribes certain norms for the maintenance and audit of budget, and accounts of such trusts and further empowers the charity commissioners to inspect and supervise the property belonging to a public trust and as well the proceedings of the trustees and books of accounts of such a trust. That apart, the act also creates certain restrictions on the investment of public trust money and as well alienation of immovable property of such a trust.

TYPES OF HOSPITALS

- *General hospital:* All establishments permanently staffed by at least two or more medical officers, which can offer in-patient accommodation and provide active medical and nursing care for more than one category of medical discipline (*e.g.* general medicine, general surgery, obstetrics).
- *Rural hospital:* Hospitals located in rural areas (classified by the Registrar General of India) permanently staffed by at least one or more physicians, which offer in-patient accommodation and provide medical and nursing care for more than one category of medical discipline (*e.g.* general medicine, general surgery and obstetrics).
- *Specialized hospital:* Hospitals providing medical and nursing care primarily for only one discipline or specific diseases (*e.g.* tuberculosis, ENT, eyes, leprosy, orthopedic, pediatrics, gynecological, cardiac, mental, cancer, infectious disease, and venereal diseases). The specialized departments, administratively attached to a general hospital and sometimes located in an annex or separate ward, may be excluded and their beds should not be considered in this category of specialized hospitals.
- *Teaching hospital:* A hospital to which a college is attached for medical/dental education.
- *Isolation hospital:* This is a hospital for the care of persons suffering from infectious diseases
- *Tertiary hospital:* States and Central Governments set up tertiary hospitals in their capitals where referred patients are treated such as AIIMS, New Delhi, P.G.I. Chandigarh, Sanjay Gandhi, P.G.I., Lucknow, etc.

CURRENT MANAGEMENT PRACTICES

Health care quality and patient safety are the common mantra of all primary and secondary health care providers. In hospitals, over the years, a variety of models and schemes for hospital interventions and development have been deployed. A typical approach is to hire external consultants to plan and implement organizational change efforts or interventions involving a wide variety of approaches.

Using the Malcolm Baldridge Award model, for example, has been a common model in hospital efforts to improve quality. One study of several of such efforts has reported mixed results. Administrators reported that they have made little progress in implementing the Baldridge quality control model or that the effort has not yet "matured".

Hospitals typically display stagnant, impersonal and historical data on various aspects of hospital performance. In one study examining the effect of change interventions in hospitals, "only 38 per cent of executives believed that their initiatives were successful and only 30 per cent thought these initiatives contributed to the sustained improvement of their organization. Also, not surprisingly, initiatives to provide training in teamwork for error reduction efforts did not result in improved outcomes.

Changing basic practices in massive, complex health care organizations will be especially challenging. However, Mohr, Burgess and Young suggest that a teamwork culture in a hospital can reduce turnover thus providing cost savings and, perhaps, higher quality service to patients.

Two realities about hospital culture and practices serve to hinder many efforts at a continuous efforts to improve patient health care outcomes. First, the status differences among providers, for example, in hospital medical/surgical wards, is often a hindrance to improved quality of service delivery and unit interpersonal communications. Physicians, of course, rightly bear all of the authority and responsibility for patient-related decisions. But physicians, because of this status, are not intimately involved in teaming with other providers when intervention efforts are undertaken.

Floor group meetings which are held by provider staff typically do not involve physicians in discussions of individual patient bedside care. When physicians make rounds to attend to patients, usually they first review medical records, view recent test data and other measures, then consult with the patient directly.

A nurse or aid is rarely consulted for face-to-face communication and, perhaps surprisingly, the physician rarely reviews nursing notes written in the patient records. The second hospital cultural factor that may hinder improvement efforts is the variation in techniques or practices caused by variations in maturity of the organization, technology used and, of course, individual differences in personality amongst hospital service providers. Such differences obviously apply to all organizations, their cultures and their practices. In a hospital, these variations often confound efforts to improve patient quality. First, the traditional model at the floor level is that when an error occurs attention is directed at identifying the cause(s) of the error. This effort, ideally, leads to correction of the error(s). Hopefully, the fix will be communicated to some personnel, but obviously not to others. When external consultants are used in an organizational development effort, these individuals are rarely familiar with internal processes and procedures.

Professionals are left to develop their own improved methods and implement them proactively, unlike the traditional "fix" model. Even threats of legal action and other environmental forces are not stimulating improvement and that the overall picture is one of randomness rather than of enlightened management.

ERROR EXAMPLES FOR ILLUSTRATION

To clarify or highlight how current medical practices and culture may negatively affect patient care quality, some examples are perhaps the best illustrator. Patients with serious medical conditions, such a cancer or other diseases that may require surgery, are often in a hospital for several weeks or months due to complications related to the foundational illness or disease process.

Patient tests and other measures are undertaken and reported in a standard routine. (Patient records are required in most cases to be kept in paper form. Some facilities also maintain duplicate records electronically.) But, a lengthy stay only increases the probability that a patient medical "error" will occur.

All of the events presented below have happened and are not fictitious:

- Patient fluids and weight are monitored but it is not unusual for a patient to gain in excess of 20 pounds before internal communication to the attending physician is executed and an IV is ordered to "fix" the problem. The aide taking the "in and out" urine measures tells the patient's caregiver, not a nurse or physician.
- Patient's lungs can gradually collapse partially before more intense respiratory therapy is ordered. Hospital cost control limits such therapy to once per day.
- The result of the above is usually a frightening experience for the patient: a breathing tube in forced down a patient's throat and their arms are tied to the bedrails so that the patient can not remove the tube.
- If they survive, after a few days, they are given a tracheotomy (another surgery) then placed on a respirator.

- A patient may go into dangerous and life-threatening shock because their white corpuscle count has been allowed to rise over a period of days, even though blood tests are given and test results provided almost daily. Infection control physicians are called in to find out the cause of the problem after the fact...if the patient lives.

Of course, not all hospital stays have the outcomes. Certainly, the cause of these and other negative outcomes can be related to human factors, technology or the catch-all "communication" problems. However, a theme that emerges here is that in each of the cases dynamics within the existing hospital culture causes the issues and could have been prevented had teamwork and communications been more fluid amongst involved service providers. The remainder of this stage will suggest a form of management development that will overcome many of the cultural factors hindering improvement in patient quality and safety. More importantly, such an initiative requires the involvement of ALL constituents in the health care arena.

SOCIO-TECHNICAL PROCESS DESIGN-TEAM DRIVEN IMPROVEMENT

Some old sayings may have some relevance here: first, "we are just too busy chopping wood to sharpen our axes" and "having lost sight of our objective, we redoubled our efforts". Teams must engage regularly in process improvement efforts as many TQM advocates have long asserted. Otherwise, they are likely repeating the same mistakes (chopping wood) without reflecting on how to do it better as a team. Also, the objective is patient care quality and safety and without reflection, care becomes its own end.

One such successful team-based programme is called socio-technical process design. To explain this seeming jargon, all work processes (patient care, surgery, sandwich factories, car making...) are both social and technical in nature.

People (the social) provide the movement of information or material (the technical) from input, to processing, and then finally to some output. Christodoulou, Babbalis and Gymnopoulos note that increasingly the need for teamwork in hospital settings is being recognized even if not sufficiently addressed in current practice.

The generic steps in socio-technical process design include

- Teams need to take time to document each step or Unit Operation in each process in which they engage. Often, a single person does one process, such as drawing blood. Also, at this stage, a physician need not be involved, but the other medical and non-medical personnel involved should be. A typical process, even sandwich making, may take 30 to 40 steps or unit operations.

- Display the steps and group or label them, *i.e.*" bread delivery and preparation."
- For each step ask the team "what can go wrong". These are called "variances" in socio-technical language. (bread is soggy) Stick to things that commonly go wrong.
- For each variance, brainstorm what can be done to prevent the variance by a technical or social solution. (Humidity can be removed with a machine or the bread could be move to a drier place or device obtained to measure humidity).
- Make changes to each step focusing on those that are easier to implement or will improve the most or same the most.
- Use all forms of communication available and even create other communication methods, if necessary, to ensure that the entire team, including the physician in the health care case, is aware of and executes the process improvements identified.
- Review other process or start from Step 1 with the process you just improved.

A natural benefit of this socio-technical process methodology include that employees are always interested in talking about their job. They know their job processes intimately and want to improve them. Also, a facilitator need not be familiar with the technical aspects of the process, only familiarity with the above steps is necessary.

Standard formats can be used for each department and process for communication or education purposes. Processes include medical information systems as well as administrative and medical records on paper. Finally, process outcomes tend to reinforce the sense of empowerment of workers to communicate key, perhaps life-saving information, to other health care personnel on a timelier basis. The current effort to create electronic data bases in health care provider organizations may be the catalyst towards which hospital management reform moves with more standardization of process and communication, resulting in organizations becoming somewhat redesigned.

To implement this move towards electronic data bases requires multi-disciplinary teams to analyse processes. Medical provider personnel as well as technology experts must necessarily be proactively involved in these efforts and the teamwork modality seems ideal for accomplishment of this function.

MEDICAL EXAMPLES

Health care processes are extremely complex and technical. Many volumes of information are produced in a hospital on a minute-by-minute basis. The usual key issues identified in health care, therefore, are how these processes are communicated, particularly if the information is unusual or indicates danger or illness for the patient.

Some examples are provided, based on observation and some of the scenarios.

- Newly empowered employees now literally put a paper flag on a record which shows an abnormal condition of a patient
- A bulletin board was created to track certain procedures, tests and other care provided to patients. Privacy was maintained since the team developed a code for both names and procedures known only to the team
- A summary form was created for key patient records such as blood count, weight or other data. The form was necessary since a patient could easily develop a 12 inch book thick medical record even after just a few weeks.
- Award and recognition system was developed and implemented with little cost, but were generated by the workers and patients themselves, not physicians or administrative personnel.
- Patients and their relatives or caregivers were give a formatted form or book similar to a diary to document events and episodes not in the record.

2

Hospital Administration and Health Supervision

HOSPITAL ADMINISTRATION

- Objective analysis and evaluation of problems and resources.
- Formation of objectives, policies, functions, and relationships.
- Organization of resources in an effective manner.
- Management through methods and means for attainment of objectives.
- Continuing evaluation and accountability.

Role Profile

- Ability to see ahead and plan accordingly; planning for the future while managing the present.
- Ability to produce and accept new and creative ideas, being an agent of change
- Willingness to take risk so as to get the new ideas accepted and implanted.
- Ability to coordinate, bringing about harmony and collaboration, organizing, allocating resources and controlling.
- Ability to delegate, making effective use of own time and that of others.
- Ability to review and evaluate, making adjustments as necessary.
- Good motivational skills to develop the people working in the hospital.

- Ability to manage stress through patience, sense of humor and a state of optimism.
- Sense of equity, fairness and social justice in all dealings within and outside the hospital.

REQUIREMENTS OF A HOSPITAL ADMINISTRATOR

Understanding the Situation: The administrator has to find out the objectives of the hospital/institution, understand the particular situation and the challenges facing it. He has to work with the people who are already there, and those who will be joining or coming by way of transfer or appointments, understand them, their motivations and aspirations and how these can be channelized to serve the objectives of the institution. These include professionals, medical, nursing and paramedical and others. He has to knit them together as a team, ignoring the groupism among the hospital staff, groups of patients, employees and public with whom he has to interact.

Integrating/Coordinating: Being the official representative of the hospital, the administrator has responsibilities for external activities like promoting a positive image of the hospital and develop good public relations with the Government, official agencies, and public at large. The hospital administrator liaises with Government and non-government organizations in developing and implementing health policies and in solving health problems of the community. He takes active interest in and encourages professional forums, publications, and educational activities.

Leading: As a leader of the organization, the hospital administrator creates a favorable organizational climate, resolves conflicts, and promotes employee morale. The hospital administrator is responsible for effective communication within the hospital-between departments and sections, hospital and its employees, and thus issues circulars and attends inter-departmental and department meetings and reports to the management on the relevant activities of the hospital.

In brief, he should have the following qualities to be an effective administrator:

- Integrity
- Self-confidence
- Decision making
- Constructive activity
- Initiative

- Enthusiasm
- Willingness to serve
- Ability to cooperate with others
- Mastery over what is happening in the hospital and healthcare in general.
- Perceptual ability-to perceive events, objectives, consequences, and implications.

Team Building: By making a cooperative effort to produce the best results by recognizing the perception of the Governing Board, colleagues, peers and the employees and by encouraging all working in the hospital in planning and carrying out the various activities. The hospital administrator has to knit together various departments in the hospital-Therapeutic, Diagnostic, and Supportive.

Knowledge, Skill and Attitude: Being the legal representative of the management, the hospital administrator is responsible for compliance by the hospital of all Government rules, legal, ethical and statutory requirements. He should have the knowledge in administrative practices-rules and regulations and must be conversant with them. He should keep himself up-to-date by continuing education leading to professional growth, positive attitude, competence and confidence.

Being Creative: Creativity is necessary to improve the functioning of any hospital and hence the hospital administrator must be creative because the situation varies from hospital to hospital. He will have to face new situations, new opportunities and new threats and he has to respond to them by initiating action or suggesting action not done before by breaking new grounds. The ability of the hospital to foster innovation and creativity often determines its success.

JOB DESCRIPTION OF A HOSPITAL ADMINISTRATOR

The administrator:

1. Administers and directs all activities of the hospital and ensures achievement of objectives in providing comprehensive healthcare, training, research, and participation of Community Health.
2. Takes all necessary steps for the maintenance of high standards-professional, technical and supportive.
3. Co-ordinates effective communication inside the hospital between departments and sections and outside the hospital with

governmental and non-governmental agencies involved in healthcare.

4. Is the transmitter, interpreter and implementer of service rules and regulations and final disciplinary authority in the hospital.
5. Delegates duties and responsibilities to appropriate persons in the hospital.
6. Prepares periodical reports including the annual report, budgetary proposals, performance reports, and audited statement of accounts.
7. Responsible for personnel policies and maintenance of accurate personnel records.
8. Monitors to the maintenance and protection of buildings, grounds and equipment.
9. Determines the need for staff and has responsibility to select, employ, confirm, grant leave, dismiss and approve salary scales in collaboration with department heads, in accordance with written rules, regulations and outlines of employee duties.
10. Oversees the acquisition of facilities and purchase of equipment and materials and ensures their proper use.
11. Understands and implements the legal requirements.
12. Implements a system to periodically review and improve the professional competence of staff through quality assurance, on-the-job training, and their continuing professional enrichment by involvement in continuing education, scientific activities and research.
13. Establishes a good system for the careful, economical and proper use of hospital finances, develop adequate financial controls, and prevent misuse of hospital funds and property.
14. Ensures that medical records are properly maintained and safeguarded.

The administrator reports to the Governing Body (or other higher authority such as Director of Health Services, Secretary to Government, etc).

Persons reporting directly to the Administrator:

- Medical Superintendent
- Nursing Superintendent
- Associate/Assistant administrators
- Co-ordinator, Community Health Programmes

- Finance Manager
- Personnel Officer

Principles of Conduct

The hospital administrator's life is dedicated to the highest possible level of performance in the competent and humane hospital care of the sick, and in pursuing this objective the hospital administrator should be guided by the following principles.

1. He will not use his position or influence for selfish personal advantage or gain and will not disparage the work of his colleagues.
2. His professional performance will be objective and fair, with the patient's best interest as the ultimate consideration.
3. The administrator will encourage, assist, and teach others the principles and practices of hospital administration to the end that future hospital administrators may be more adequately prepared.
4. In his relationships with the medical staff of the hospital he will support that which is constructive, sound, and in the interests of good hospital professional practices. He will resist and oppose that which is, in his judgment, harmful, destructive or unwise.
5. The administrator will seek constantly to improve his professional knowledge and skill and will accept counsel and guidance, particularly in the fields with which he is not entirely familiar.
6. In his relationships with personnel and staff he will be impartial, tolerant, fair and interested in all reasonable means of promoting personnel morale and welfare, consistent with the hospital's best interests and ability to provide them.
7. Recognizing that his is a position of public trust, he will, within the limitation imposed by good judgment, legal considerations, and his hospital charter respect the rights, privileges, and beliefs of others regardless of race, colour, or creed. When his administrative duties bring him into conflict with any segment of society or belief, he will deal with the situation with the greatest consideration, courtesy, and respect for the individual that is possible, without any ridicule or animosity.

The hospital administrator plays a vital a role in saving lives, without having to take scalpel in hand. Hospital administrators manage hospitals, outpatient clinics, hospices, and drug-abuse treatment centers. In large hospitals, there may be several administrators, one for each department.

In smaller facilities, they oversee the day-to-day operations of all departments. Administrators make sure hospitals operate efficiently and provide adequate medical care to patients. Their responsibilities are numerous and sometimes require the assistance of the medical and support staff.

They act as liaisons between governing boards, medical staff, and department heads and integrate the activities of all departments so they function as a whole. Following policies set by a governing board of trustees, administrators plan, organize, direct, control and coordinate medical and health services. Administrators recruit, hire, and sometimes train doctors, nurses, interns, and assistant administrators. Administrators plan budgets and set rates for health services. In research hospitals, administrators develop and expand programs and services for scientific research and preventive medicine. In teaching hospitals, they aid in the education of new doctors. Administrators plan departmental activities, evaluate doctors and other hospital employees, create and maintain policies, help develop procedures for medical treatments, quality assurance, patient services, and public relations activities such as active participation in fund-raising and community health planning. Hospital administrators work long or irregular hours. Hospitals are open round the clock – 24/7 – and administrators may be called in at any hour to make decisions and resolve disputes. Administrators also attend staff meetings, participate in health planning councils, go to fund-raising events, and travel to professional association conventions. A hospital administrator's job is difficult and demanding. They need to keep up with advances in medicine, computerized diagnostic and treatment equipment, data processing technology, government regulations, health insurance changes, and financing options. While doctors strive to keep the blood flowing and the heart beating, the hospital administrator is doing his job in keeping the hospital alive and healthy.

HEALTH SUPERVISION

Turner syndrome, as used in this report, refers to a condition characterized by short stature and ovarian digenesis in females who have a single X chromosome and absence of all or part of the second sex chromosome (X or Y). No chromosomal gonad digenesis is excluded. The birth prevalence of Turner syndrome has been estimated to be from 1 in 2000 to 1 in 5000 female live births. Approximately 1% to 2% of all concept uses have a 45,X chromosome constitution.

The majority (99%) of these spontaneously abort, usually during the first trimester of pregnancy. With the more frequent use of ultrasonography, it is recognized that some pregnancies with a fetal 45,X chromosome constitution progressing into the second trimester are associated with uncial cysts, severe lymph edema, or hydrous fetal is. These pregnancies are associated with a high frequency of fetal death.

Phenotype

Pediatricians are most familiar with the clinical findings that prompt the diagnosis of Turner syndrome in children, namely, short stature and other features, such as lymph edema, webbed neck, low posterior hairline, and cubits values. A wide range of clinical abnormalities, including cardiac and renal anomalies, may be found (Table 1). Turner syndrome, however, is not always accompanied by distinctive features and most often is not diagnosed in infancy.Later in childhood, Turner syndrome maybe suspected primarily because of short stature. Other prominent presenting features in teenage years are delayed puberty and delayed menarche, and in adult women, an ovulation and infertility.

Growth in children with Turner syndrome is characterized by a slight intrauterine growth restriction, slow growth duringinfancy and childhood, and lack of a pubertal growth spurt.Because of delayed epiphyseal closure, small gains in height may occur even after 20 years of age. Average height is rarely achieved, except in girls with mosaicism (the presence in an individual of 2 or more chromosomally different cell lines, both originating from the same zygote) or those whose parents are of above average height. The anticipated adult height is approximately 143 cm and rarely exceeds 150 cm.

Although intelligence is normal, individuals with Turner syndromeare at risk of impairments in the cognitive, behavioral, and social domains. These include learning disabilities, particularly with regard to spatial perception, visual-motor integration, mathematics, memory, the ability to formulate goals and plan action sequences to attain them, and attention span.As a result, the nonverbal IQ in persons with Turner syndrome tends to be lower than the verbal IQ. The behavioral abnormalities differ by age. Younger girls may be hyperactive, immature, and anxious, and anxiety, depression, and unsatisfactory peer relationships are more common in older girls.

A female with 45,X Turner syndrome may manifest an X-linked recessive disorder, such as hemophilia, because she has only 1 X chromosome. Therefore, when an X-linked disorder is identifiedin a female, the possibility of Turner syndrome caused by monotony X (absence of an X chromosome: 45,X) or a structural abnormality of an X chromosome should be considered.

Cytogenetics

Most characteristics of Turner syndrome appear to result from haploinsufficiency of specific genes on the X chromosome, although abnormal pairing of the sex chromosomes during meiosis is the major factor in acolyte loss and gonadal digenesis. Haploinsufficency refers to the presence in the cell of 1 set of genes rather than the usual 2 sets. In 46,XX female embryos, inactivation of 1 X chromosome, referred to as lionization, occurs in every somatic cell shortly after fertilization. Some genes involved in Turner syndrome, however, seem to escape inactivation. Thus, the 46,XX female embryo has a functional diploid set of these "pseudo-autosomal" genes. These genes also seem to have homology on the Y chromosome, which accounts for the normal growth and development in XY male embryos.

Current evidence indicates that the genes involved in Turnersyndrome are mainly located on the short arm of the X chromosome: X. A distal homeobox gene (SHOX),* located in the pseudoautosomal region of the X chromosome (PAR1), has been shown to contribute to short stature and some of the skeletal abnormalities observed in individuals with Turner syndrome. Haploinsufficency of this gene has been associated with Leri-Weillsyndrome, an osteochondrodysplasia characterized by short stature, mesomelic dwarfism, Madelung deformity, and other skeletal abnormalities. Loci contributing to normal ovarian function and fetal viability have been identified on the long arm of the X chromosome.

In approximately 80% of girls with 45,X Turner syndrome, the single remaining X chromosome is inherited from the mother, and in 20% of these girls, it is inherited from the father. Imprinting (an alteration in the expression of a gene or a chromosome, depending on whether the genetic material is inherited from the mother or father) does not seem to operate, because the phenotype of an individual with 45,X Turner syndrome does not vary according to the parental origin of the X chromosome.A recent study identified a putative imprinted X-linked gene related to cognitive function, but this has not yet been confirmed.When the diagnosis of Turner syndrome is suspected, the appropriate test for confirmation is chromosome analysis.

A wide range of karyotypic abnormalities exists within Turner syndrome. When conventional karyotyping is performed using lymphocyte cultures, about 50% of patients show a 45,X chromosome constitution. Another karyotype found with Turner syndrome is mosaicism of 45,X with other cell lines, such as 46,XX, 46,XY, or 47,XXX.

Although mosaicism with a 46,XX line (which is the most frequent mosaicism found with 45,X) tends to result in a subtler phenotype on average,the clinical findings cannot be predicted in an individual case. Structural anomalies of an X chromosome, such as isochromosomes (an abnormal chromosome with equal arms originating from a transverse division of the centromere during cell division, instead of the normal longitudinal division), deletions, rings, or translocations,also may be found in a person with Turner syndrome. Structural X anomalies are often mosaic with 45,X or 46,XX cells.

Mosaicism in individuals with Turner syndrome may be more common than was previously thought. When 2 tissues (lymphocytes and fibroblasts) were examined, approximately 80% of patients with 45,X Turner syndrome were found to have mosaicism.[27] Mosaicism in live-born girls with Turner syndrome is more common than that in fetuses with Turner syndrome, suggesting that a second sex chromosome (or a critical portion of a second sex chromosome) may be necessary for fetal survival and that most, or perhaps all, individuals with Turner syndrome have mosaicism. A Y chromosome is present in 5% to 6% of individuals with Turner syndrome, and an additional 3% have a marker chromosome (a structurally abnormal chromosome that cannot be identified by conventionalcytogenetic methods) derived from either the Y or another chromosome.

Girls with 45,X Turner syndrome should have an adequate cytogenetic examination for covert Y chromosome mosaicism, including fluorescence in situ hybridization. Routine use of polymerase chain reaction to identify cryptic Y chromosomal material is not recommended. However, when the karyotype shows a marker chromosome of unknownorigin, molecular studies using Y chromosome DNA probes may be helpful in the diagnosis. The possibility of Y chromosomemosaicism also should be investigated thoroughly if clitoromegaly or masculinized genitalia are present at birth or if virilization occurs at puberty.When Y chromosome mosaicism is present, there is an increased risk, estimated from 7% to 10%, for developing gonadoblastoma or dysgerminoma in the dysgenetic gonads, andprophylactic gonadectomy is recommended.

Buccal smears for X chromatin bodies (Barr bodies) should not be used to screen for or diagnose Turner syndrome. They do nothave sufficient sensitivity and specificity, because individuals with mosaicism or a structural X abnormality are often X chromatin positive. Also, a Y chromosome would not be detected in a routine buccal smear that only looks for X chromatin bodies.

Medical treatment

Short Stature

Growth hormone (GH) therapy is standard care for a child with Turner syndrome and is usually begun after the child'sheight falls below the fifth percentile for healthy girls in the same age cohort. More than one half of girls with Turnersyndrome will have fallen below the fifth percentile by 2 years of age. For those who experience early growth failure, it appears reasonable to begin GH therapy as early as 2 years of age. A multicenter study of the efficacy and safety of GH initiated at even earlier ages is currently being conducted. Biosynthetichuman GH increases the rate of growth in most girls with Turner syndrome without advancing the bone age. Some reports indicate increases in final adult height of 8 to 10 cm if they receive at least 6 years of GH therapy and estrogen production is delayed.Greater height gains have recently been achieved even without delaying estrogen production by initiating GH at an early age and at high doses.

Cardiovascular Abnormalities

The prevalence of cardiovascular abnormalities among patients with Turner syndrome varies in different series between 20% and 40%. It is higher in patients with monosomy X than in those with structural abnormalities of the X chromosome and in girls with a more pronounced clinical phenotype, such as those with congenital lymphedema and webbed neck, than in those with milder clinical manifestations. Cardiovascular abnormalities typically involve the left side of the heart. Bicuspid aortic valve is the most common malformation, followed by coarctation of the aorta. Other less common but still significant cardiovascular defects in individuals with Turner syndrome are mitral valve prolapse, partial anomalous pulmonary venous drainage, and hypoplastic left heart syndrome.

Many of these malformations result in an increased susceptibility to endocarditic, and therefore, prophylactic administration of antibiotics before dental or surgical procedures is essential. Aortic root dilatation, present in 3% to 8% of patients with Turner syndrome, may lead to dissecting aneurysm, rupture, and death. Although in most cases aortic dilatation precedes recognized aortic dissection, not all cases end in dissection and not all cases of dissection have antecedent aortic root dilatation. Bicuspid aortic valve, forestation of the aorta, and systemic hypertension has been identified in approximately 90% of patients with aortic dilatation and dissection.These are the same risk factors that are associated with aortic root dilatation in the general population.

However, because of the current lack of knowledge about the natural history of aortic dilatation, additional research will be required to identify the best strategy for timely discovery of the problem. In the absence of naturalhistory data, some authorities would advise aortic arch imaging of such patients by echocardiogram or magnetic resonance imaging (MRI) as frequently as every 3 years. Although most instances of aortic dilatation or dissection in individuals with Turner syndrome have been reported among adults, reports of its occurrence in females 21 years or younger raise the possibility that surveillance imaging of the aortic arch for young patients with Turner syndrome could be valuable.

The observation of cystic medial necrosis in individuals with aortic root dilatation has led some to postulate that the aortic abnormality may be caused by a mesenchymal defect. This contention is supported by the evidence of other connective tissue abnormalities, such as those involving the skeletal and lymphatic systems, in patients with Turner syndrome.

On the basis of these considerations, it is recommended that, as part of the initial evaluation, all patients with Turnersyndrome have a baseline cardiology evaluation. This may include an echocardiogram, preferably performed at a centre experienced in pediatric cardiology, because data indicate that more than one half of echocardiograms performed in children at facilities mostly devoted to adult studies are technically not adequate for interpretation.

The schedule and nature of the cardiology follow-up should be directed by the pediatric cardiologist in concert with the primary care pediatrician and individualized to the patient's needs and the type of defect(s) identified.

Patients with bicuspid aortic valve, aortic stenosis, coarctation of the aorta, or systemic hypertension need close follow-up for aortic dilatation. The cardiologist should decide the periodicity of the evaluations and the method of appraisal (MRI versus echocardiography). Although echocardiography is considered the mainstay of diagnosis, MRI can detect dilatation missed on echocardiography.

In addition, MRI should be used when aortic root dilatation is detected to evaluate its severity and provide more precise measurements for follow-up, when findings on echocardiography are equivocal, and when there are technical difficulties because of chest wall configuration or obesity. MRI also can be valuable in assessing the possibility of aortic dissection.

In patients in whom the cardiology evaluation during childhood is normal, the primary care pediatrician should pay special attention to the cardiovascular examination, including blood pressure, peripheral pulses, and murmurs. Although there are no evidence-based data regarding the need for a follow-up cardiology evaluation, some have proposed a repeat cardiologic examination during adolescence, ideally performed by a pediatric cardiologist, to look for asymptomatic aortic dilatation.

Primary care pediatricians and pediatric cardiologists need to be aware of the risk of aortic dissection and educate their patients with Turner syndrome about the signs and symptoms of this complication.

Although there has been reassurance that GH does not cause cardiac hypertrophy in girls without cardiac malformation, there is inadequate information about its use in girls with underlying aortic stenosis, with or without underlying bicuspid aortic valve.

Hypertension

Up to 40% of girls with Turner syndrome have hypertension,and when identified, it should be treated vigorously. Although in most cases hypertension is idiopathic, a careful search for cardiovascular or renal causes should be made.

Hearing Loss

Hearing loss is common in individuals with Turner syndrome. Recurrent otitis media occurs in most girls with Turner syndrome. In addition, a progressive infrequency sensor neural hearing loss often occurs, which neccesitates the use of hearing aids in some children and more than 25% of women by their mid-forties.

Strabismus

The incidence of strabismus is markedly increased in girls with Turner syndrome, developing in about one third between the ages of 6 months and 7 years. Anterior chamber abnormalities are also more common in girls with Turner syndrome than in those without and may present as congenital glaucoma.

Craniofacial Anomalies

If craniofacial anomalies cause concern, consider plastic surgery for the neck, face, or ears before the child enters school or thereafter, as indicated. Some individuals with Turner syndrome have a tendency to form keloids, which must be taken into account when surgery is considered.

Obesity

Because obesity may be a problem in girls with Turner syndrome, diet and exercise for weight control should be discussed.

Glucose Intolerance

Glucose intolerance occurs more frequently in persons with Turner syndrome than in the general population; however, diabetes mellitus seems to be rare.[52,55] Monitoring of fasting blood glucose concentrations should be considered in girls who are significantly overweight, have a strong family history of type 2 diabetes mellitus, are Hispanic or African American, or have signs of insulin resistance, such as acanthosis nigricans.

Urinary Tract Abnormalities

Approximately one third of patients with Turner syndrome have a structural malformation, most commonly horseshoe kidneys, a double collecting system, or abnormal vascular supply. Although most of these malformations do not have clinical significance, they may result in an increased risk of hypertension, urinary tract infections, or hydronephrosis.

Thyroid Dysfunction and Other Autoimmune Disorders

Autoimmune disorders that appear to be more prevalent in individuals with Turner syndrome than the general population include Hashimoto thyroiditis, celiac disease, inflammatory bowel disease, and juvenile rheumatoid arthritis. Individuals with Turner syndrome are at especially high risk of developing hypothyroidism, but this rarely occurs before 4 years of age.

Orthopedic Problems

Congenital developmental dysplasia of the hip occurs more frequently in girls with Turner syndrome than in the general population.This contributes to the development of arthritis of the hips in older individuals. Girls with Turner syndrome also have an increased risk of scoliosis, kyphosis, and lordosis.

Psychosocial Support

The primary care pediatrician should 1) review the psychologicsupport available to the child and family to optimize the child's psychosocial adjustment; 2) encourage family support by referral to other individuals with Turner syndrome, parents of children with Turner syndrome, or a Turner syndrome support group; and 3) supply the family with literature on Turner syndrome.

The Prenatal Visit

When a prenatal diagnosis of 45,X Turner syndrome or another karyotype associated with Turner syndrome is detected, counseling is ordinarily provided for the family by a medical geneticist, a pediatric endocrinologist, or another physician with special knowledge of Turner syndrome. Sometimes, because of a previous relationship with the family, the pediatrician may be asked to review the information and to assist the family in decision making.

Turner syndrome may be diagnosed or suspected prenatally because of ultrasonographic evidence of fetal edema or nuchal cystic hygroma. Ultrasonography showing a left-sided cardiac defect, renal anomalies, growth retardation, or relatively short limbs also may suggest Turner syndrome. A Turner syndrome karyotype may be discovered fortuitously when fetal chromosome analysis is performed for reasons not associated with an increased incidence of Turner syndrome, such as advanced maternal age. Karyotyping performed when the results of maternal serum screening with multiple markers (maternal serum α-fetoprotein, human chorionic gonadotropin, and unconjugated estriol) project an increased risk for Down syndrome also has detected some fetuses with Turnersyndrome.If an abnormality associated with Turner syndrome is diagnosed by ultrasonography or if multiple marker screening is positive, the recommended follow-up is fetal karyotyping using amniotic fluid cells obtained by amniocentesis or fetalblood obtained by percutaneous umbilical blood sampling when the karyotype is needed more rapidly.

The spectrum of clinical findings cannot be predicted from the fetal karyotype alone, even in nonmosaic 45,X Turner syndrome. The variability may be increased by mosaicism, which is often not detected in the fetal chromosome analysis. A diagnosis of Turner syndrome made solely by fetal karyotyping should be followed up with careful ultrasonography to define the phenotypic abnormalities as accurately as possible.

Most instances of mosaicism of 45,X and 46,XY diagnosed prenatally have been associated with phenotypically healthy male newborn infants, although the possibility of some clinical abnormality later in life cannot be excluded. If a 45,X or 46,XY fetal karyotype is found, ultrasonographic examination is helpful in diagnosing normal-appearing male genitalia. Determination of amniotic fluid follicle-stimulating hormone (FSH) and testosterone concentrations also may be helpful in confirming the male phenotype.

ANTICIPATORY GUIDANCE

The pediatrician should discuss the diagnosis of Turner syndrome, the phenotype, and the variability of the phenotype. Both parents should be present if possible.

They need to know that short stature and infertility are likely, mental retardation is unlikely, some congenital anomalies may be present, and some learning difficulties are expected for most but not all individuals. Discuss the treatments and interventions available, such as growth-enhancing therapy and sex hormone replacement, and emphasize that with medical supervision and psychosocial counseling and support, girls with Turner syndrome may lead healthy, satisfying lives. In cases of early prenatal diagnosis, however, some parents may decide to terminate the pregnancy.

Most often, Turner syndrome is a sporadic event, and the risk of recurrence is not increased for subsequent pregnancies. There may be some rare exceptions, however, such as inheritance of a structural X anomaly and inherited mosaicism.

Health Supervision From Birth to 1 Month of Age: Newborn

- Confirm the diagnosis of Turner syndrome and review the karyotype. If a prenatal diagnosis was made, discuss with the geneticist whether further cytogenetic studies should be performed. Chromosome analyses from peripheral blood or other tissue samples may be indicated, depending on the adequacy of the prenatal study and the possibility of mosaicism, especially for the Y chromosome. Evaluate the child for typical features of Turner syndrome as follows.

- Examine the child's hips for dysplasia. Repeat the examination several times during early infancy.
- Review results of the newborn hearing screening.
- Obtain an initial consultation with a cardiologist with experience in pediatric cardiology for all persons with Turner syndrome. This includes patients who had "normal" results on prenatal ultrasonographic examination, because bicuspid aortic valve or coarctation could have been missed.
- Check blood pressure and peripheral pulses during each physical examination. A careful comparison of arm and leg systolic pressure is important to evaluate for possible coarctation.
- Perform a renal ultrasound (or repeat the ultrasound if it was done prenatally). If the patient is found to have an abnormality of the urinary tract, continue monitoring for urinary tract infections and renal function.
- Distinguish the anomalies having major implications on the medical treatment (eg, cardiac and renal anomalies) from those of primarily cosmetic and psychologic importance.
- Inform the family that lymphedema may persist for months or longer and may recur.
- Discuss the possibility of feeding problems. Some infants with Turner syndrome have inefficient sucking and swallowing reflexes because of impaired oral motor function.
- Obtain an initial consultation with a pediatric endocrinologist to discuss the current status of endocrine therapy for growth and for the development of secondary sex characteristics. Indicate that infertility is almost always present, although assisted reproduction techniques may enable infertile women with Turner syndrome to have children.
- Discuss subacute bacterial endocarditis prophylaxis if a cardiac anomaly is present.
- Talk about how and what to tell other family members and friends.

Health Supervision From 1 Month to 1 Year of Age: Infancy

- Assess the infant's weight, taking into account that many infants wfant to developmental intervention programs if neuromuscular development is delayed.

Health Supervision on From 1 TO 5 Years of Age: Early Childhood

- Follow the child's growth and have her evaluated by a pediatric endocrinologist if growth failure occurs. The age at which GH therapy is initiated varies but can be considered at as early as 2 to 3 years of age for girls who are below thefifth percentile for height in the growth chart for healthy girls of the same age. Early initiation of GH therapy may allow for greater gain and normalization of the timing of puberty. Plot growth on the Turner syndrome-specific growth curve starting at 2 years of age (Fig).
- Evaluate the child's speech and refer the child to a speech therapist when appropriate. Consider hearing loss as a possible cause of speech delay.
- If a cardiac anomaly is present, have the patient followed up as recommended by her cardiologist.
- Check blood pressure and peripheral pulses during each physical examination. A careful comparison of arm and leg systolic pressure is important to evaluate for possible coarctation.
- Evaluate the child's hearing and check for serous otitis and otitis media during every visit.
- Continue to evaluate the child's renal status (urinalysis and culture, as indicated) if a renal anomaly is present.
- Test for thyroid function by measuring thyroid-stimulating hormone and free or total thyroxine levels at 1- to 2-year intervals because of the increased frequency of hypothyroidism usually caused by autoimmune thyroiditis. In the absence of clinical signs, initiation of thyroid function testing may be delayed until after 4 years of age or later, because hypothyroidism is rare before then.
- Evaluate the child for possible developmental delay and learning difficulties, particularly spatial perception problems. An assessment of the child before entering a preschool programme may benefit the child and parents as well as schoolpersonnel. Information about testing and evaluation resources may be obtained from the school or from state and regional programs for persons with developmental disabilities.
- If hypertension is present, treat it aggressively and performa careful search for cardiovascular or renal causes.

- Counsel the parents regarding environmental factors that may increase the risk of otitis media, such as bottle feeding, passive smoking, and group child-care facility attendance. If otitis media is present, institute aggressive treatment. Discuss the option of tympanostomy tubes for persistent otitis media and consider referral to an otolaryngologist.

Health Supervision From 5 TO 13 Years of Age: Late Childhood

- Discuss the diagnosis and treatment of Turner syndrome with the child as soon as she is able to understand as well as with the parents.
- Continue to monitor growth carefully. In addition to GH, the endocrinologist may consider adding oxandrolone to the GH treatment regimen in older girls (9–12 years of age) with extreme short stature or those in whom the response to GH is not adequate.
- Monitor the child for urinary tract infections if urinary tract abnormalities are present.
- Check blood pressure and peripheral pulses during each physical examination. A careful comparison of arm and leg systolic pressure is important to evaluate for possible coarctation.
- Evaluate the child's hearing and check for serous otitis and otitis media during every visit. Advise patients to protect their hearing by avoiding loud noises.
- Check the child's dentition for malocclusion.
- Continue testing for thyroid function at 1- or 2-year intervals.
- Check for scoliosis yearly. Lordosis and kyphosis are also seen more frequently in girls with, than in girls without, Turner syndrome.
- Watch for potential school problems, such as specific learning disabilities, attention deficits, hyperactivity, and difficulty in developing social skills. Refer the child for educational evaluation and intervention, as indicated. Encourage parents to interact with school personnel.
- Discuss adjustment to short stature with the parents and separately with the child.
- If hypertension is present, treat it aggressively and perform a careful search for cardiovascular or renal causes.

- If otitis media is present, institute aggressive treatment. Discuss the option of tympanostomy tubes for persistent otitismedia and consider referral to an otolaryngologist. Advise patients to protect their hearing by avoiding loud noises.
- Counsel the family regarding the importance of optimizing bone density, and advise that the patient receive the recommended daily requirements for Vitamin D and calcium through diet or supplementation.

HEALTH SUPERVISION FROM 13 TO 21 YEARS OR OLDER: ADOLESCENCE TO EARLY ADULTHOOD

- Examine the adolescent for pigmented nevi, which may not be prominent in young children but tend to increase in frequency in adolescence and older ages. Pigmented nevi have primarilycosmetic significance. Advise removal of the nevi if they are rubbed by clothing. The risk of melanoma, which is low, does not appear to be increased by GH treatment.
- Check blood pressure and peripheral pulses during each physical examination. A careful comparison of arm and leg systolic pressure is important to evaluate for possible coarctation.
- Measure fasting lipid profile at least once during adolescence to screen for hyperlipidemia, especially in those who have a positive family history, have diabetes mellitus, or are overweight.
- Evaluate the child's hearing and check for serous otitis and otitis media during every visit. If otitis media is present,institute aggressive treatment. Advise patients to protect their hearing by avoiding loud noises.
- Check the adolescent annually for scoliosis and kyphosis.
- Even for individuals with normal initial cardiac evaluation, refer to a cardiologist for a complete evaluation, including a close evaluation of the aortic root.
- Continue to test the adolescent's thyroid function every 1 to 2 years.
- Evaluate the adolescent for development of secondary sex characteristics. As many as one third of girls with mosaicism will enter puberty spontaneously. Measurement of luteinizing hormone (LH) and FSH concentrations may be helpful in assessing gonadal function.[70] Increased LH and FSH concentrations will help to

confirm that the child is physiologically ready for initiation of estrogen therapy, and evidence of suppression of LH and FSH into the normal range may help to determine adequacy of the maintenance dose chosen.

- Refer the adolescent to a pediatric endocrinologist for evaluation of sex hormone replacement. If gonadotropin levels are increased, initiate estrogen therapy and then begin cyclic therapy with a progestin at an appropriate age. Estrogen therapy may be initiated as early as 12 years of age for girls who are satisfied with their height. For others, estrogen therapy can be delayed until as late as 15 years of age to maximize height. Individualize treatment choices concerningthe timing of feminizing therapy and length of growth enhancing therapy to the patient's psychosocial needs.
- If hypertension is present, treat it aggressively and performa careful search for cardiovascular or renal causes.
- If otitis media is present, institute aggressive treatment.
- If lymphedema is exacerbated by estrogen therapy, combined decongestive therapy that uses manual lymphatic drainage, low-stretch support garments, and exercises may be effective.[71] Some physicians also use diuretics.
- Continue to monitor school function and behaviour.
- Discuss social adaptation. Girls with Turner syndrome tend to be socially immature for their age and need support in developing independence and social interactions. Support groups of girls with Turner syndrome are especially helpful. Provide psychosexual counseling.
- Present information on reproductive options to bearing children, such as adoption and medically assisted reproduction.
- Provide counseling regarding sexuality and sexually transmitted diseases.
- Refer the rare girl with Turner syndrome who has sufficient ovarian function to ovulate and who may become pregnant for genetic counseling and prenatal diagnosis (if pregnant). These girls are at increased risk of having a fetus with chromosome abnormalities and having miscarriages. Offer contraception advice when appropriate.
- Facilitate transfer of the adolescent to adult medical care.

NURSING CARE OF THE HOSPITALIZED CHILD

The most common reasons for hospitalization of children remain acute illnesses or injuries and exacerbations of chronic illnesses or conditions. Great importance continues to be placed on limitingthe duration of hospitalization and use of inpatient resources. Patients with less serious problems may be admitted for observation or short stays. Patients are discharged from inpatient units as soon as they can be appropriately cared for and their ongoing needs can be met on an outpatient basis.

Although hospital costs may be decreased as a result, a shortened stay should not curtail a thorough evaluation and treatment course. Given these circumstances, the attending physician has an essential role in ensuring that the hospitalized child receives appropriate and comprehensive care that is appropriately continued on an outpatient basis. Such continuous care is a fundamental feature of health care delivered within a child's medical home.

As the care that is delivered on an outpatient or short-stay basis becomes more sophisticated, illnesses of hospitalizedchildren are becoming more complex and severe and frequently require subspecialty consultation. Although the primary care physician may be the attending physician directly responsible for clinical management of the hospitalized child, this is not always the case. In community hospitals, pediatric sub specialists may be unavailable, anda physician whose primary practice is adult medicine may provide subspecialty and surgical care and function as attending physician for pediatric patients. Alternatively, a full-time teaching attending physician, specialist, or designated hospitality may be responsible for the supervision and care of the child.[2] In no case should the primary care physician be denied the opportunity to participate in the clinical care of the patient.

Coordination and oversight of care must be provided by the appropriate physician(s) caring for the patient, whether that be the primary care physician or another physician(s) as described above. The following functions are the essential components of this coordination and oversight role. Each of these activities contributes materially to the care of the patient and warrants reimbursement, regardless of the specific physician(s) performing the function.

Initial Assessment

For any child requiring hospital admission, an initial assessment made before or at the time of hospitalization allows for the child to be admitted to the inpatient setting that is best suited to his or her specific problem(s). If the inpatient or hospital setting best suited to the child's needs is not on the approved list of the child's insurance carrier, the physicians caring for the child must advocate for the best interest of the child and seek approval for admission to the appropriate setting.

A complete evaluation includes a history of the present illness; past medical history; pain assessment; review of systems; review of immunizations; assessment of growth, developmental, educational, and emotional status; review of family and social history, including review of behavioral and environmental risk factors; and a physicalexamination.[4]The effects of the child's condition on his or her family and the effects of the family on the child's condition need to be evaluated to initiate family-centered care. These assessments may be performed just before or concurrent with hospitalization and routinely involve collaboration with other nonphysician health care professionals, such as nursingstaff, child life specialists, social workers, etc.

Obtaining History From The Primary Care Physician

It is especially important that the child's medical history be obtained when the primary care physician is not the primaryattending physician. Hospital-based attending physicians, surgeons, and subspecialists who hospitalize children with complex or multiple problems must communicate with the child's primary care physician for overall coordination of care.

If necessary, this may include obtaining authorization for specific services. For children with new onset of acute problems, preexisting illness, chronic disease, and/or past hospitalizations, hospital andoutpatient information must be available on admission for the inpatient health care team to review. Access to this informationprevents unnecessary duplication of previous diagnostic and therapeutic measures, allows primary care and hospital-basedphysicians to update the status of past conditions that may not be obvious on the current admission, provides insight into psychosocial issues facing the patient and family, and facilitates monitoring the child's growth and development.

Additionally, this information may indicate that a condition initially considered appropriate for a short-stay unit actually requires formal inpatient hospitalization. Inpatient and outpatient facilities must to be able to provide and receive necessary medical records in a reliable, timely, safe, and confidential manner.

Ongoing Role Of The Primary Care Physician

When physicians other than the primary care physician participate in the care of the child, the primary care physician can help ensure continuity of care and help the family develop trust in providers who have no preexisting relationship with the family. When the primary care physician does not directly participate in hospital-based care, regular communication with the attending physician enables the primary care physician to remain actively involved in the patient's care. As the hospitalization progresses, the primary care physician can provide valuable insight into the patient's changing medical condition and the patient's and family's psychosocial status and response.

The primary care physician can help integrate and coordinate the input of various physicians when multiple consultants are involved in the patient's care. The continued involvement of the primary care physician ensures discharge planning is proceeding effectively. It improves the primary care physician's understanding of the patient's hospital course to facilitate optimal transitional and ongoing outpatient care. For patients and families facing end-of-life issues, the involvement of the primary care physician is particularly valuable.

Pediatric Consultation For Adult Subspecialists And Surgeons

When the attending physician does not routinely care for pediatric patients, pediatric consultation can help with the physiologic, pharmacologic, and psychosocial issues unique to younger and smaller patients. The patient's primary care physician may fill this clinical role. Alternatively, another general pediatrician, or family practitioner with demonstrated consistent experience in the inpatient care of children may serve as a consultant. Such formal consultation is particularly recommended for any hospitalized child with complex medical or psychosocial problems and all patients who are younger than 14 years or less than 40 kg in body weight.

Discharge Plans And Coordination

Before discharge, an assessment of the child's needs should be made, plans should be formulated, treatment should be provided, and necessary information should be supplied to family members. Treatment plans must be made in accordance with the child's developmental, educational, and emotional level. Family members or guardians must be involved with formulation of the treatment plan, because they are ultimately responsible for decisions about the care their child receives.

If treatment is not completed during hospitalization, appropriate outpatient management must be arranged. The child's social, developmental, and family status are particularly important,because most children will receive part of their treatment on an outpatient basis. The attending physician, together with other members of the health care team and the family, is responsible for evaluating whether the outpatient treatment plan appears feasible for the child's family to undertake and modifying the plan if needed. At the time of discharge, a written summary and recommendations for outpatient care must be available to all personnel and institutions involved in the future care of the child.

Timely dictation services should be available to ensure a complete and legible record of events is provided. Laboratory, imaging, and consultative reports pending at the time of discharge should be specifically identified. Referrals must be provided for all needed outpatient services, including a source of primary care if the child does not have a primary care physician. In such instances or when the primary care physician was not directly involved in the child's hospitalization,the provider responsible for ongoing care should be contacted directly by the inpatient team before the day of discharge to ensure continuity of care. All referrals for outpatient services should be arranged with providers familiar with the special needs of children.

Occasionally the child's physicians, when determining the need for inpatient care, may not be in agreement with decisions made by external organizations (eg, review organizations or health maintenance organizations or insurance companies). Standards of medical care established by peer groups should be used as guidelines when controversy exists with the understanding that the guidelines may not be applicable to each child's situation. In such instances, as in all instances, treatment and discharge decisions must be made with the best interest of the child as the primary motivation.

3

Hospital Service and Management

Hospitals are not merely profit making organizations, more over they have the responsibility of taking care of human health. Since they provide prestigious service, they have a higher value in the society. In order to maintain that value, hospitals must take utmost care in providing health care services. Proper co- ordination of resources like man, machine, money and material is required to maintain superior quality in services rendered. The Enterprise Resource Planning (ERP) tool called Hospital Information System developed by Dewsoft Solutions is an ideal package for integrating an entire healthcare organization. We serve you better, because we know you better.

Healthcare providers usually face the challenge of minimizing cost without compromising the quality of services. Since hospitals are concerned with the life of the patients, any small error can lead to an irrecoverable loss - we know these facts better than anyone else, that's why utmost care is taken in preparing this ERP solution for hospitals.

ORGANIZATIONAL STRUCTURE OF A HOSPITAL

Objectives/Rationale

Every hospital, large or small, has an organizational structure that allows for the efficient management of departments.

Key Points

Power Point: Importance of Understanding Organizational Structure of Hospital;

A. facilitates the understanding of the hospital's chain of command
B. shows which individual or department is accountable for each area of the hospital

Complexity of Organizational Structure Depends on Size of Healthcare Facility; large acute care hospitals have complicated structures, whereas, the smaller institutions have a much simpler organizational structure;

Grouping of Hospital Departments Within the Organizational Structure;

A. Although each hospital department performs specific functions, departments are generally grouped according to similarity of duties.

B. Departments are also grouped together in order to promote efficiency of the healthcare facility.

C. Common organizational categories might include:

1. Administration Services (often referred to simply as "administration")
2. Informational Services
3. Therapeutic Services
4. Diagnostic Services
5. Support Services (sometimes referred to as "Environmental Services")

Administration Services—business people who "run" the hospital.

A. Hospital Administrators

1. manage and oversee the operation of departments
   a. oversee budgeting and finance
   b. establish hospital policies and procedures
   c. perform public relation duties
2. generally include: Hospital President, Vice Presidents, Executive Assistants, Department Heads

Informational Services—documents and process information;

A. Admissions-often the public's first contact with hospital personnel

1. checks patients into hospital
   a. responsibilities include: obtaining vital information (patient's full name, address, phone number, admitting doctor, admitting diagnosis, social security number, date of birth, all insurance information)
   b. frequently, admissions will assign in house patients their hospital room .

Therapeutic Services – provides treatment to patients;

A. includes the following departments:

1. Physical Therapy (PT)
   a. provide treatment to improve large-muscle mobility and prevent or limit permanent disability
   b. treatments may include: exercise, massage, hydrotherapy, ultrasound, electrical stimulation, heat application
2. Occupational Therapy (OT)
   a. goal of treatment is to help patient regain fine motor skills so that they can function independently at home and work
   b. treatments might include: arts and crafts that help with hand-eye coordination, games and recreation to help patients develop balance and coordination, social activities to assist patient's with emotional health
3. Speech/Language Pathology
   a. identify, evaluate, and treat patients with speech and language disorders
   b. also help patients cope with problems created by speech impairments
4. Respiratory Therapy (RT)
   a. treat patient's with heart and lung diseases
   b. treatment might include: oxygen, medications, breathing exercises
5. Medical Psychology
   a. concerned with mental well-being of patients
   b. treatments might include: talk therapy, behavior modification, muscle relaxation, medications, group therapy, recreational therapies (art, music, dance)
6. Social Services
   a. aid patients by referring them to community resources for living assistance (housing, medical, mental, financial)
   b. social worker specialties include: child welfare, geriatrics, family, correctional (jail)
7. Pharmacy
   a. dispense medications per written orders of physician, dentists, etc.
   b. provide information on drugs and correct ways to use them
   c. ensure drug compatibility

8. Dietary - responsible for helping patients maintain nutritionally sound diets
9. Sports Medicine
   a. provide rehabilitative services to athletes
   b. teaches proper nutrition
   c. prescribe exercises to increase strength and flexibility or correct weaknesses
   d. apply tape or padding to protect body parts
   e. administer first aid for sports injuries
10. Nursing (RN, LVN, LPN)
    a. provide care for patients as directed by physicians
    b. many nursing specialties include: nurse practitioner, labor and delivery nurse, neonatal nurse, emergency room nurse, nurse midwife, surgical nurse, nurse anesthetist
    c. In some facilities, *Nursing* is a service in and of itself.

Diagnostic Services – determines cause(s) of illness or injury;

A. includes the following departments:
   1. Medical Laboratory (MT) - studies body tissues to determine abnormalities
   2. Imaging
      a. image body parts to determine lesions and abnormalities
      b. includes the following: Diagnostic Radiology, MRI, CT, Ultra Sound
   3. Emergency Medicine - provides emergency diagnoses and treatment

Support Services—provides support to entire hospital;

A. includes the following departments:
   1. Central Supply
      a. in charge of ordering, receiving, stocking and distributing all equipment and supplies used by healthcare facility
      b. sterilize instruments or supplies
      c. clean and maintain hospital linen and patient gowns
   2. Biomedical Technology
      a. design and build biomedical equipment (engineers)
      b. diagnose and repair defective equipment (biomedical technicians)

c. provide preventative maintenance to all hospital equipment (biomedical technicians)
d. pilot use of medical equipment to other hospital employees (biomedical technicians)

3. Housekeeping and Maintenance
   a. maintain safe clean environment
   b. cleaners, electricians, carpenters, gardeners

EVOLUTION OF THE INTERNATIONAL NETWORK OF HEALTH PROMOTING HOSPITALS

In order to support the introduction of health promotion programmes in hospitals, the WHO Regional Office for Europe started the first international consultations in 1988. In the subsequent year, the WHO model project "Health and Hospital" was initiated with the hospital Rudolfstiftung in Vienna, Austria, as a partner institution. After this phase of consultation and experimenting the HPH movement went into its developmental phase, being marked by the initiation of the European Pilot Hospital Project by the WHO Regional Office for Europe in 1993. This phase, which lasted from 1993 to 1997, involved intensive monitoring of the development of projects in 20 partner hospitals from 11 European Countries.

Subsequent to the closing of this pilot phase, national and regional networks were developed and the network reached its consolidation phase. Since then, national and regional networks take an important role in encouraging the cooperation and exchange of experience between hospitals of a region or a country, including the identification of areas of common interest, the sharing of resources and the development of common evaluation systems. In addition, a thematic network exists, bringing together psychiatric hospitals and allowing the exchange of ideas and strategies in this particular field. The International Network of Health Promoting Hospitals acts as a network of networks linking all national/regional networks. It supports the exchange of ideas and strategies implemented in different cultures and health care systems, developing knowledge on strategic issues and enlarging the vision. As of May 2005, the International HPH Network comprises 25 Member States, 35 national and regional networks and more than 700 hospitals. As defined in the WHO Health Promotion Glossary, *"Health promotion* evaluation is an assessment of the extent to which health promotion actions achieve a *'valued' outcome".* Assessment methods and outcomes differ in health promotion as compared to clinical medicine.

With the current focus of health system and hospital managers on outcomes, qualitative methods are frequently considered as offering only weak evidence. In fact, the longterm benefit of many health promotion interventions makes it necessary to distinguish between different levels of health promotion outcomes, beyond changes in clinical parameters and in health status. In the context of health promotion participation, partnership, empowerment and actions directed to the creation of supportive environments are also important aspects that need to be evaluated, and many proponents of health promotion indeed recommend different levels of analysis. Don Nutbeam suggests distinguishing outcomes according to health promotion outcomes, intermediate outcomes and health and social outcomes:

- *Health promotion outcomes* refer to modifications of personal, social and environmental factors to improve people's control over the determinants of health (e.g. health literacy, social influence and action, healthy public policy and organizational culture);
- *Intermediate outcomes* refer to changes in the determinants of health (e.g. lifestyles, access to health services, reduction of environmental risks);
- *Health and social outcomes* refer to subjective (self reported assessments such as Nottingham Health Profile, SF-36 or EUROQOL) and objective measures (weight, cholesterol level, blood pressure measurement, biochemical test, mortality) of changes in health and in social status (e.g. equity).

The HPH movement has provided many good examples of health promotion interventions that hospitals can carry out. Some of these interventions have been evaluated in the literature as being highly effective and cost-effective as described in the chapter on Evidence for Health Promotion in this volume. Some may discard the narrow view of health promotion activities that were evaluated using controlled designs, and argue that our understanding goes beyond these activities.

Activities in Health Promoting Hospitals

Currently, the quality of health promoting activities in the hospitals of the International HPH network is not systematically assessed. Hospitals becoming members of the International Network:

- endorse the fundamental principles and strategies for implementation of the Vienna Recommendations;
- belong to the National/Regional HPH Network in the countries where such networks exist (hospitals in countries without such networks apply directly to the international coordinating institution); and
- comply with the rules and regulations established at the international and national/regional levels.

Hospitals in the International Network further have to commit themselves to become a smoke-free hospital and to run three specific projects/activities addressing health issues of staff, patients, community, or improving organizational routines with a possible impact on health. A web-based database has been established to register projects and activities, providing information on key indicators of the hospital and on health promotion activities.

At the international level, attempts have been made to review and develop evaluation systems for health promotion. The Fourth and Fifth Annual Workshop of National and Regional Network Coordinators in 1998 and 1999 addressed the issue and concluded that so far, evaluations, if any, were mostly carried out at project level, only a few strategies of quality assurance were applied at network level and most coordinators experienced great problems in developing and applying evaluation schemes. There are different evaluation approaches at national and regional network levels, although none of them are well developed yet.

Among the most developed tools applied was the Hospital Accreditation Scheme that evolved from the Healthy Hospital Award in the United Kingdom. Hospitals were formally accredited as Health Promoting Hospital after application, standardized self-audit survey and external assessment to validate the survey and interview staff and patients.

A similar system was installed in the German system consisting of two peer-reviews from hospitals and one site-visit from a representative of the network to the applicant hospital. External assessors decided on the acceptance in the network. However, the German experience shows that, due to the financial implications, these visits are difficult to carry out. The German Network has also worked on adapting the excellence model of the European Foundation of Quality Management and the Balanced Scorecard for the systematic implementation of health promotion in the hospitals' organizational structure and culture. A report on the process of this work is also available in the present volume.

In 1994, the Polish Network started a self-assessment system to monitor the improvement of individual hospital performance; however, its application was not continued due to validity and reliability issues of the tool. The Danish Network decided in December 2000 to initiate the establishment of a set of standards; part of this work is also presented in this volume.

Other countries in the WHO European Region initiated in the past similar schemes consisting of site-visits, peer review, self-assessment, and surveys. Outside Europe, the Ministry of Health in Thailand conducted a survey comparing 17 Health Promoting Hospitals with 23 non-HPH. A questionnaire was designed and items were constructed for a self-assessment of HPH strategy implementation according to the following dimensions: a) Leadership and administration, b) Resource allocation and Human Resource development, c) Supportive environment, d) Health promotion for staff, e) Health promotion of patients and families, and f) Community health promotion. Many methodological issues need to be resolved before a valid comparison can be made; however, the survey contains many innovative ideas that may be elaborated in the future.

EVIDENCE-BASED HEALTH PROMOTION IN HOSPITALS

While "curative" medicine is delivered to symptomatic patients who seek health care, health promotion and preventive interventions will often attempt to modify individuals' lives, and this must be based on the highest level of randomized evidence "that our preventive manoeuvre will do more good than harm".

Practice guidelines are considered valid if "when followed, they lead to the health gains and the costs predicted for them", and they must be based on evidence from trials using valid methods. Evidence is usually categorized as:

1a: Evidence from meta-analysis of randomized controlled trials;

1b: Evidence from at least one randomized controlled trial;

2a: Evidence from at least one controlled study without randomization;

2b: Evidence from at least one other type of quasi-experimental study;

3: Evidence from descriptive studies, such as comparative studies, correlation studies and case-control studies;

4: Evidence from expert committee reports or opinions or clinical experience of respected authorities, or both.

Health promotion should be based on a high level of evidence, i.e. level 1a, 1b or 2a, whenever possible. Weaker evidence may be used for describing good clinical practice in health promotion in hospitals, but whenever category 1a to 2a is absent, it should be considered relevant to establish new evidence. Clinical trials in the spectre of health promotion must meet the same criteria for quality as other randomized trials. They are: Appropriateness of inclusion and exclusion criteria, concealment of allocation, blinding of patients and health professionals if possible, objective or blind method of data collection, valid or blind method of data analysis, completeness and length of follow up, appropriateness of outcome measures and statistical power of results.

The large group of qualitative studies are outside the evidence definition. They describe the opinions and feelings of selected persons, and they are based upon the specific interviewer's interpretation and competences, and the concrete context. They are important for an implementation process and may give rise to new hypothesis, but the results can seldom be generalized. Using both quantitative research and qualitative studies is a unique combination in exploring new areas for investigation and implementation.

Concepts Used

In public health, disease prevention is usually defined as a) primary disease prevention which prevents diseases from occurring, b) secondary prevention which detects disease at an early stage and prevents disease from developing, and c) tertiary prevention or rehabilitation which prevents aggravation or recurrence of disease and secures maintenance of functional level.

Traditionally, hospitals primarily take care of tasks that relate to secondary or tertiary prevention whereas the primary sector and other social institutions take care of primary prevention. It is, however, increasingly recognized that also hospitals can play a significant role in primary prevention. When integrating health promotion in clinical activity it makes more sense to use a classification that distinguishes between patient pathways in ordinary clinical practice, staff and the community:

- Patients: General health promotion which should be offered to all patients and which addresses all patient pathways. Specific health promotion vis-a-vis defined patient groups, characterized through their belonging to certain diagnosis groups or otherwise.

- Staff: General health promotion aiming at a healthy and safe work environment. Training in the field of clinically related health promotion.
- Community: Cooperation with relevant structures and organizations.

General health promotion addresses general determinants of health and disease (including tobacco, alcohol, nutrition, physical activity and psychosocial issues). One example of this is lifestyle intervention, which involves activities aiming to influence individual behaviour (alcohol consumption, smoking etc.). Lifestyle intervention includes counselling, recommendations and empowering the patients to enhance their competence and their capability.

Specific health promotion addresses conditions that are significant for specific patient groups. Examples of this are the prevention of complications in diabetes patients, education of asthma patients, cardiac rehabilitation etc. An important element in disease-related health promotion is strengthening the patient's ability to manage his/her condition.

Policy of Health Promotion in Hospitals

Hospitals are a special type of workplace with many employees that are exposed both physically and mentally in connection with their clinical tasks. In spite of work environment regulations, many exposures and risk situations cannot be avoided. Therefore it is necessary for hospitals to have a health promotion policy. On the basis of existing knowledge of the importance of lifestyle factors for treatment and prognosis, all hospitals should establish policy, counselling services, education and support for health promotion as an integrated part of the individual patient pathway as well as for the staff.

Effect of a health promotion policy in hospitals is based upon descriptive studies, exclusively, giving a low level of evidence.

Health Promotion for Hospital Staff

Those working in the health care sector can play an important role in promoting health, either through providing examples of what can be done to achieve a healthy environment or through using their authority to act as advocates for public health policies or in giving advice to individual patients or citizens.

Learning and teaching in methods used in health promotion and patient education should build on evidence. The individual lifestyle habits of health care staff, their attitudes and competencies influence the way they handle prevention issues.

Staff who are smokers generally underestimate the role of smoking as a risk factor, whereas non-smokers in some cases overestimate this risk factor. Thus smokers are less prone to advise patients on lifestyle issues in general and the same is true of staff that feel that they have too little training in this field. Staff who are smokers do not convey through their behaviour the health knowledge they are supposed to communicate to the patients; there is a cognitive disparity between their behaviour and their knowledge, i.e. staff either choose to stop smoking or ignore their knowledge to the detriment of advice for patients.

Interestingly, staff that stops smoking initiate more interventions among patients with improved effect. Special competences are another important way of improving the integration in the clinical daily life. The implementation rates are given for "spontaneous" motivational counselling in the emergency department, for the usual staff, and for specialist nurses in three successive periods, each including 100 patients. Specialized staff offer more systematic advice on smoking cessation than other staff.

EMPOWERMENT OF PATIENTS FOR HEALTH PROMOTING MANAGEMENT OF CHRONIC ILLNESS

Expert interventions in hospitals provide in general only a turning point in disease processes, and a basis for recuperation or the successful management of chronic illness. The main part of recuperation or of the day-to-day illness management (prevention of aggravation, negative long-term effects, social consequences etc.) has to be performed primarily by the patients themselves – with specific professional support by the hospital, specialized services, the family doctor or other health care services and lay support. This phase of the illness career lasts much longer and is out of direct control of the hospital, but is crucial for the outcome of regaining health and quality of life.

Professional support for this phase is in its core educative: primarily information, consultation, and training.

Hospitals have to take this mid-range perspective on the illness career into account by either providing necessary disease specific support by themselves or by referring patients to other, specialized providers in the health care system. The more complex and the more rare the disease and its treatment gets, the more likely it remains a task of the hospital itself, but this of course requires adequate legal and financial regulation which allows to provide these services systematically. Within the International HPH network, there are many examples of effective interventions of this type of services, e.g. diabetes training, COPD training.

Empowerment of Patients for Health Promoting Lifestyle Development

The health gain of hospital interventions can be even further increased when taking on a more long term perspective. Future health can be improved by lifestyle changes – thus reducing disease-related risks and developing positive health potentials and resources. It is primarily educative services (information, consultation, training) that can be utilized to influence individual lifestyles. These types of services can be offered by different providers, e.g. other providers in health care, social services and adult education.

Hospitals are in a good position to offer such services, having already developed a relationship with patients in a crisis situation, being centres of knowledge and having a high prestige in the area of health. Health education can become a module in a package of educational communication, using the opportunity of the relationship and the time in the hospital. Investments in this direction would help to develop hospitals into genuine health centres.

HOSPITALS: ORGANIZATIONAL STRUCTURE AND QUALITY MANAGEMENT

More than a decade ago, the WHO Health Promoting Hospitals (HPH) project was initiated in order to support hospitals towards placing greater emphasis on health promotion and disease prevention, rather than on diagnostic and curative services alone. The Health Promoting Hospitals strategy focuses on meeting the physical, mental and social needs of a growing number of chronically ill patients and the elderly; on meeting the needs of hospital staff, who are exposed to physical and psychological stress; and on meeting the needs of the public and the environment.

Twenty hospitals in eleven European countries participated in the European pilot project from 1993 to 1997. Since then, the International Network of Health Promoting Hospitals has steadily expanded and now covers 25 Member States, 36 national or regional networks and more than 700 partner hospitals.

But, what has been achieved with regard to the implementation of health promotion services at both hospital and network level? What is the scope of health promotion activities in hospitals and how can the principles laid out in the Ottawa Charter for Health Promotion be put into practice? Is there an evidence base for health promotion and has this facilitated the expansion of health promotion services in hospitals? Is health promotion a service anyway? How does health promotion relate to quality management? And how can we evaluate the quality of health promotion activities in hospitals?

HOSPITAL SERVICES

Inpatient hospital services are defined in Title XVIII of the Social Security Act and in the regulations:

- Subject to the conditions, limitations, and exceptions set forth in this subpart, the term "inpatient hospital or inpatient CAH services" means the following services furnished to an inpatient of a participating hospital or of a participating CAH or, in the case of emergency services or services in foreign hospitals, to an inpatient of a qualified hospital:
  - Bed and board.
  - Nursing services and other related services.
  - Use of hospital or CAH facilities.
  - Medical social services.
  - Drugs, biologicals, supplies, appliances, and equipment.
  - Certain other diagnostic or therapeutic services.
  - Medical or surgical services provided by certain interns or residents-intraining.
  - Transportation services, including transport by ambulance.
- Inpatient hospital services does not include the following types of services:
  - Posthospital SNF care, as described in 42 CFR 409.20, furnished by a hospital or a critical access hospital that has a swing-bed approval.
  - Nursing facility services, described in 42 CFR 440.155 that may be furnished as a Medicaid service under title XIX of the Act in a swing- bed hospital that has an approval to furnish nursing facility services.

- Physician services that meet the requirements of 42 CFR 415.102(a) for payment on a fee schedule basis.
- Physician assistant services, as defined in §1861(s)(2)(K)(i) of the Act.
- Nurse practitioner and clinical nurse specialist services, as defined in §1861(s)(2)(K)(ii) of the Act.
- Certified nurse mid-wife services, as defined in §1861(gg) of the Act.
- Qualified psychologist services, as defined in §1861(ii) of the Act.
- Services of an anesthetist, as defined in 42 CFR 410.69.

Blood must be furnished on a day which counts as a day of inpatient hospital services to be covered and to count towards the blood deductible. Thus, blood is not covered under and does not count towards the blood deductible when furnished to an inpatient after the inpatient has exhausted all benefit days in a benefit period, or where the individual has elected not to use lifetime reserve days.

However, where the patient is discharged on their first day of entitlement or on the hospital's first day of participation, the hospital is permitted to submit a billing form with no accommodation charge, but with ancillary charges including blood. The records for all Medicare hospital inpatient discharges are maintained in CMS for statistical analysis and use in determining future PPS DRG classifications and rates.

Non-PPS hospitals do not pay for non-covered services generally excluded from coverage in the Medicare Programme. This may result in denial of a part of the billed charges or in denial of the entire admission, depending upon circumstance.

In PPS hospitals, the following are also possible:

- In appropriately admitted cases where a non-covered procedure was performed, denied services may result in payment of a different DRG (*i.e.*, one which excludes payment for the non-covered procedure); or
- In appropriately admitted cases that become cost outlier cases, denied services may lead to denial of some or all of an outlier payment.

The following examples illustrate this principle. If care is non-covered because a patient does not need to be hospitalized, the intermediary denies the admission and makes no payment unless paid under limitation on liability. Under limitation on liability, Medicare payment may be made when the provider and the beneficiary were not aware the services were not necessary and could not reasonably be expected to know that he services were not necessary.

If a patient is appropriately hospitalized but receives only non-covered care, the admission is denied:

- *NOTE:* The intermediary does not deny an admission that includes covered care, even if non-covered care was also rendered. Under PPS, Medicare assumes that it is paying for only the covered care rendered whenever covered services needed to treat and/or diagnose the illness were in fact provided.

If a non-covered procedure is provided along with covered non-routine care, a DRG change rather than an admission denial might occur. If non-covered procedures are elevating costs into the cost outlier category, outlier payment is denied in whole or in part.

When the hospital is included in PPS, most of the subsequent discussion regarding coverage of inpatient hospital services is relevant only in the context of determining the appropriateness of admissions, which DRG, if any, to pay, and the appropriateness of payment for any outlier cases. If a patient receives items or services in excess of, or more expensive than, those for which payment can be made, payment is made only for the covered items or services or for only the appropriate prospective payment amount. This provision applies not only to inpatient services, but also to all hospital services under the programme.

If the items or services were requested by the patient, the hospital may charge him the difference between the amount customarily charged for the services requested and the amount customarily charged for covered services.

An inpatient is a person who has been admitted to a hospital for bed occupancy for purposes of receiving inpatient hospital services. Generally, a patient is considered an inpatient if formally admitted as inpatient with the expectation that he or she will remain at least overnight and occupy a bed even though it later develops that the patient can be discharged or transferred to another hospital and not actually use a hospital bed overnight.

The physician or other practitioner responsible for a patient's care at the hospital is also responsible for deciding whether the patient should be admitted as an inpatient. Physicians should use a 24-hour period as a benchmark, *i.e.*, they should order admission for patients who are expected to need hospital care for 24 hours or more, and treat other patients on an outpatient basis.

However, the decision to admit a patient is a complex medical judgement which can be made only after the physician has considered a number of factors, including the patient's medical history and current medical needs, the types of facilities available to inpatients and to outpatients, the hospital's by-laws and admissions policies, and the relative appropriateness of treatment in each setting.

Factors to be considered when making the decision to admit include such things as:

- The severity of the signs and symptoms exhibited by the patient;
- The medical predictability of something adverse happening to the patient;
- The need for diagnostic studies that appropriately are outpatient services (*i.e.*, their performance does not ordinarily require the patient to remain at the hospital for 24 hours or more) to assist in assessing whether the patient should be admitted; and
- The availability of diagnostic procedures at the time when and at the location where the patient presents.

Admissions of particular patients are not covered or non-covered solely on the basis of the length of time the patient actually spends in the hospital.

In certain specific situations coverage of services on an inpatient or outpatient basis is determined by the following rules:

- Minor Surgery or Other Treatment - When patients with known diagnoses enter a hospital for a specific minor surgical procedure or other treatment that is expected to keep them in the hospital for only a few hours (less than 24), they are considered outpatients for coverage purposes regardless of: the hour they came to the hospital, whether they used a bed, and whether they remained in the hospital past midnight.
- Renal Dialysis - Renal dialysis treatments are usually covered only as outpatient services but may under certain circumstances be covered as inpatient services depending on the patient's condition. Patients staying at home, who are ambulatory, whose conditions are stable and who come to the hospital for routine chronic dialysis

treatments, and not for a diagnostic workup or a change in therapy, are considered outpatients. On the other hand, patients undergoing short-term dialysis until their kidneys recover from an acute illness (acute dialysis), or persons with borderline renal failure who develop acute renal failure every time they have an illness and require dialysis (episodic dialysis) are usually inpatients. A patient may begin dialysis as an inpatient and then progress to an outpatient status.

Under original Medicare, the Quality Improvement Organization (QIO), for each hospital is responsible for deciding, during review of inpatient admissions on a case-by-case basis, whether the admission was medically necessary. Medicare law authorizes the QIO to make these judgements, and the judgements are binding for purposes of Medicare coverage.

In making these judgements, however, QIOs consider only the medical evidence which was available to the physician at the time an admission decision had to be made. They do not take into account other information (*e.g.*, test results) which became available only after admission, except in cases where considering the post-admission information would support a finding that an admission was medically necessary.

ACCOMMODATIONS – GENERAL

The programme will pay the same amount for routine accommodations services whether the patient has a private room not medically necessary, a private room medically necessary (Medicare does not pay for deluxe accommodations in any case), a semiprivate room (2-, 3-, or 4-bed accommodations), or ward accommodations, if its ward accommodations are consistent with programme purposes.

A provider having both private and semiprivate accommodations may nevertheless charge the patient a differential for a private room if:

- The private room is not medically necessary; and
- The patient (or relative or other person acting on their behalf) has requested the private room, and the provider informs them of the amount of charge at the time of the request.

The private room differential may not exceed the difference between the customary charge for the accommodations furnished and the most prevalent semiprivate accommodation rate at the time of the patient's admission. Where the provider bills for a private room as a covered service, *i.e.*, shows the charge for the room as a covered charge on the Form CMS-1450, the intermediary will deem the private room to be medically necessary.

Where the provider, on the other hand, shows a private differential as a non-covered charge, the intermediary will assume that the private room is not medically necessary. If the beneficiary (or their representative) protests a charge for the private room on the grounds that the privacy was medically necessary, such protest will, if not in written form, be reduced to writing and forwarded to the intermediary.

The intermediary will then develop the facts and make a specific determination regarding the medical necessity of the private room. (If an intermediary receives many protests of this kind, the provider may need guidance on what constitutes medical necessity for privacy).

If the protest is received after the claim is processed, it will be treated as a request for reconsideration. If at any time in the course of development (or thereafter within the period when the determination is not administratively final), the provider acknowledges that the private room was medically necessary; the intermediary will make an immediate finding to this effect.

Medical Necessity - Need for Isolation

A private room is medically necessary where isolation of a beneficiary is required to avoid jeopardizing their health or recovery, or that of other patients who are likely to be alarmed or disturbed by the beneficiary's symptoms or treatment or subjected to infection by the beneficiary's communicable disease.

For example, communicable diseases, heart attacks, cerebra-vascular accidents, and psychotic episodes may require isolation of the patient for certain periods.. In establishing the medical necessity for isolation, the date of the physician's written statement is not controlling, nor is the presence of a written statement.

The crucial question is whether a private room was ordered by the physician because it is necessary for the health of the patient himself or herself or of other patients.

In the absence of such an order, a patient who requested the room with knowledge of the amount of the charge may be charged appropriately, even though a physician subsequently submits a statement that the room was medically necessary.

There may be cases in which the physician's written statement of medical necessity, though dated after admission or even after discharge, merely confirms an order made informally at or before the time the beneficiary was admitted to the private room (*e.g.*, the physician made arrangements by phone for the patient's admission, gave the diagnosis, and stated the beneficiary would need a private room).

In such cases, assuming that the private room was medically necessary, the lack of a written statement by the physician, or the fact that the written statement was prepared after discharge, would not be controlling. The patient may not be charged.

Medical Necessity - Admission Required and Only Private Rooms Available

A private room is considered to be medically necessary even though the beneficiary's condition does not require isolation if he/she needs immediate hospitalization (*i.e.*, the beneficiary's medical condition is such that hospitalization cannot be deferred) and the hospital has no semiprivate or ward accommodations available at the time of admission.

It need not be considered whether semiprivate or ward accommodations were available in some other accessible hospital. Where medical necessity exists, the provider may not charge the beneficiary a private room differential until semiprivate or ward accommodations become available.

Thereafter the provider may transfer the patient to the non-private accommodations, or allow them to continue occupancy of the private room, subject to an appropriate differential charge if they request the private room with knowledge of the amount of the charge. If the admission could be deferred until semiprivate or ward accommodations become available, the beneficiary should be informed of the amount of the differential he/she must pay for a private room if he/she wishes to be admitted immediately.

The beneficiary may be charged the specified differential if he/she has been admitted to the private room at their request (or at the request of their representative) with knowledge of the amount of the charge.

Charges for Deluxe Private Room

Beneficiaries found to need a private room (either because they need isolation for medical reasons or because they need immediate admission when no other accommodations are available) may be assigned to any of the provider's private rooms. They do not have the right to insist on the private room of their choice, but their preferences should be given the same consideration as if they were paying all provider charges themselves.

The programme does not, under any circumstances, pay for personal comfort items. Thus, the programme does not pay for deluxe accommodations and/or services. These would include a suite, or a room substantially more spacious than is required for treatment, or specially equipped or decorated, or serviced for the comfort and convenience of persons willing to pay a differential for such amenities.

If the beneficiary (or representative) requests such deluxe accommodations, the provider should advise that there will be a charge, not covered by Medicare, of a specified amount per day (not exceeding the differential defined in the next sentence); and may charge the beneficiary that amount for each day he/she occupies the deluxe accommodations. The maximum amount the provider may charge the beneficiary for such accommodations is the differential between the most prevalent private room rate at the time of admission and the customary charge for the room occupied.

Beneficiaries may not be charged this differential if they (or their representative) do not request the deluxe accommodations.

The beneficiary may not be charged such a differential in private room rates if that differential is based on factors other than personal comfort items. Such factors might include differences between older and newer wings, proximity to lounge, elevators or nursing stations, desirable view, etc.

Such rooms are standard 1-bed units and not deluxe rooms for purposes of these instructions, even though the providor may call them deluxe and have a higher customary charge for them. No additional charge may be imposed upon the beneficiary who is assigned to a room that may be somewhat more desirable because of these factors.

All Private Room Providers

If the patient is admitted to a provider which has only private accommodations, and no semiprivate or ward accommodations, medical necessity will be deemed to exist for the accommodations furnished. Beneficiaries may not be subjected to an extra charge for a private room in an all-private room provider.

Wards

The law contemplates that Medicare patients should not be assigned to ward accommodations except at the patient's request or for a reason consistent with the purposes of the health insurance programme. When ward accommodations are furnished at the patient's request or for a reason determined to be consistent with the program's purposes, payment will be based on the average per diem cost of routine services. Where ward accommodations are assigned for other reasons, the law provides what may be a substantial penalty. Any request by the patient (or relative or other person responsible for his or her affairs) for ward accommodations must be obtained by the provider in writing and kept in its files.

Assignment Consistent With Programme Purposes

It is considered to be consistent with the program's purposes to assign the patient to ward accommodations if all semiprivate accommodations are occupied, or the facility has no semiprivate accommodations. However, the patient must be moved to semiprivate accommodations if they become available during the stay. Some hospitals have a policy of placing in wards all patients who do not have private physicians. Such a practice may be consistent with the purposes of the programme if the intermediary determines that the ward assignment inures to the benefit of the patient.

In making this determination, the principal consideration is whether the assignment is likely to result in better medical treatment of the patient (*e.g.*, it facilitates necessary medical and nursing supervision and treatment). The intermediary should ask a provider having this policy to submit a statement describing how the assignments are made, their purpose, and the effect on the care of patients so assigned. If the intermediary makes a favourable determination on a practice affecting all ward assignments of Medicare patients in the institution, a reference should be made on the appropriate billing form for patients to whom the hospital assigned a ward pursuant to such practice.

Assignment Not Consistent With Programme Purposes

It is not consistent with the purposes of the law to assign a patient ward accommodation based on their social or economic status, their national origin, race, or religion, or their entitlement to benefits as a Medicare patient, or any other such discriminatory reason. It is also inconsistent with the purposes of the law to assign patients to ward accommodations merely for the convenience or financial advantage of the institution. Additionally, under DRGs, there no longer is a reduction to payment or an adjustment to the end of year settlement.

Charges

Customary charges means amounts which the hospital or skilled nursing facility is uniformly charging patients currently for specific services and accommodations. The most prevalent rate or charge is the rate that applies to the greatest number of semiprivate or private beds in the institution.

NURSING AND OTHER SERVICES

Nursing and other related services, use of hospital facilities, and medical social services ordinarily furnished by the hospital for the care and treatment of inpatients are covered under hospital insurance and included in the Prospective Payment system payment.

- *NOTE:* The services of a private-duty nurse or other private-duty attendant are not covered. Private-duty nurses or private-duty attendants are registered nurses, licensed practical nurses, or any other trained attendant whose services ordinarily are rendered to, and restricted to, a particular patient by arrangement between the patient and the privateduty nurse or attendant. Such persons are engaged or paid by an individual patient or by someone acting on their behalf, including a hospital that initially incurs the costs and looks to the patient for reimbursement for such non-covered services.

Where the hospital acts on behalf of a patient, the services of the private-duty nurse or other attendant under such an arrangement are not inpatient hospital services regardless of the control which the hospital may exercise with respect to the services rendered by such private-duty nurse or attendant.

Anesthetist Services

If the hospital engages the services of a nurse anesthetist or other non-physician anesthetist (either on a salary or fee-for-service basis) under arrangements which provide for billing to be made by the hospital, the cost of the service when provided to an inpatient could be covered.

Medical Social Services to Meet the Patient's Medically Related Social Needs

Medical social services are services which contribute meaningfully to the treatment of a patient's condition.

Such services include, but are not limited to:

- Assessment of the social and emotional factors related to the patient's illness, need for care, response to treatment, and adjustment to care in the facility;
- Appropriate action to obtain case work services to assist in resolving problems in these areas; and
- Assessment of the relationship of the patient's medical and nursing requirements to their home situation, financial resources, and the community resources available to them in making the decision regarding their discharge.

DRUGS AND BIOLOGICALS

Drugs and biologicals for use in the hospital, which are ordinarily furnished by the hospital for the care and treatment of inpatients, are covered.

Three basic requirements must be met for a drug or biological furnished by a hospital to be a covered hospital service:

- The drug or biological must represent a cost to the institution in rendering services to the beneficiary;
- The drug or biological must meet the statutory definition. Under the statute, payment may be made for a drug or biological only where it is included, or approved for inclusion, in the latest official edition of the United States Pharmacopoeia-National Formulary (USP-NF), the United States Pharmacopoeia Drug Information (USP DI), or the American Dental Association (ADA) Guide to Dental Therapeutics, except for those drugs and biologicals unfavourably evaluated in the ADA Guide to Dental Therapeutics. Combination drugs are also included in the definition of drugs if the combination itself or all of the therapeutic ingredients of the combination are included, or approved for inclusion, in any of the above drug compendia. Drugs and biologicals are considered approved for inclusion in a compendium if approved under the established procedure by the professional organization responsible for revision of the compendium; or be approved by the pharmacy and drug therapeutics or equivalent committee of the medical staff of the hospital for use in the hospital.

Drugs or biologicals approved for marketing by the Food and Drug Administration (FDA) are considered safe and effective for purposes of this last requirement when used for indications specified in the labeling.

Therefore, use of an FDA-approved drug or biological is covered if:

- It was administered on or after the date of the FDA's approval;
- It is reasonable and necessary for the individual patient; and
- All other applicable coverage requirements are met.

Drugs and biologicals, which have not received final marketing approval by the FDA, are not covered unless CMS instructs the intermediary to the contrary. However, FDAapproved drugs are used for indications other than those specified on the labeling. As long as the FDA has not specified such use as non-approved, coverage is determined taking into consideration the generally accepted medical practice in the community. For example, the labeling of certain chemotherapeutic drugs indicates their use in the therapy of specified types of cancer. However, based on experience and empirical evidence, physicians may prescribe these drugs for a wider range of cancer treatments than what is indicated in the labeling.

Local medical review policy may or may not grant coverage, depending on the circumstances. Determinations as to whether use of a drug or biological is reasonable and necessary for an individual patient are the responsibility of the Quality Improvement Organization (QIO), if this is stage of the review for a PPS acute care admission.

However, if this is an excluded service claim being reviewed by the intermediary, the intermediary reviews and makes a determination, unless it cannot and needs to refer it to the QIO for an initial determination. A hospital stay solely for the purpose of use of a drug or biological that is determinod not reasonable and necessary is not covered.

Drugs Included in the Drug Compendia

Medicare covers only those drugs and biologicals included, or approved for inclusion, in the latest official edition or revision of the compendia as previously listed. Where a drug is excluded from coverage because it is unfavourably evaluated in either the AMA Drug Evaluations or Accepted Dental Therapeutics, the exclusion applies to all uses for which the drug or biological was so unfavourably evaluated. Drugs and biologicals are considered "approved for inclusion" in a compendium if approved under the procedure established by the professional organization responsible for revision of the compendium.

Approval by Pharmacy and Drug Therapeutics Committee

A pharmacy and drug therapeutics or equivalent committee is a medical staff committee that confers with the hospital pharmacist in the formulation of policies pertaining to drugs. Drugs and biologicals approved for use in the hospital by such a committee are covered only if the committee develops and maintains a formulary or list of drugs accepted for use in the hospital.

The committee need not function exclusively as a pharmacy and drug therapeutics committee but may also carry on other medical staff functions. Drugs and biologicals are considered approved for use in the hospital if selected for inclusion in the hospital drug list of formulary under the procedure of the committee established for that purpose.

Express approval is required; the fact that a drug or biological has not been specifically determined to be unacceptable for use in the hospital does not constitute approval. Drugs and biologicals are covered if approved for general use in the hospital, or if approved for use by a particular patient or group of patients.

Approval by a pharmacy and drug therapeutics committee is an alternative to approval for inclusion of the drug or biological in an approved drug compendium; such approval does not preclude the need for a determination of medical necessity. An investigational drug is not considered to meet the reasonable and necessary test since its efficacy has not yet been established.

The decision of individual hospitals should not transcend the determinations of the Food and Drug Administration and Public Health Service in respect to the safety and effectiveness of drugs. Therefore, even if approved by an appropriate hospital committee, the reasonable cost of an investigational or other non-approved drug or biological (*e.g.*, Laetrile) cannot be reimbursed.

This exclusion from payment applies whether or not the drug or biological is administered during the course of an otherwise covered hospital stay, since payment may not be made for items and services that are not reasonable and necessary.

A hospital stay solely for the purpose of administering a drug or biological that is not reasonable and necessary, including an investigational drug or biological, is not covered and the drug or biological itself is not covered.

Combination Drugs

Combination drugs are covered if the combination itself or all of the therapeutic ingredients of the combination are included, or approved for inclusion, in any of the designated drug compendia. Any combination drug approved for use in the hospital by the pharmacy and drug therapeutics or equivalent committee is covered.

Drugs Specially Ordered for Inpatients

Coverage is not limited to drugs and biologicals routinely stocked by the hospital; a drug or biological not stocked by the hospital, which the hospital obtains for the patient from an outside source, such as a community pharmacy, can also be covered. Drugs and biologicals not included in the drug list or formulary maintained by the hospital's pharmacy and drug therapeutics committee may be covered if the hospital has a policy which permits such drugs to be furnished to a patient at the special request of a physician. However, in order to be covered, such drugs and biologicals must be included, or approved for inclusion, in one of the designated drug compendia.

Drugs for Use Outside the Hospital

Drugs and biologicals furnished by a hospital to an inpatient for use outside the hospital are, in general, not covered as inpatient hospital services. However, if the drug or biological is deemed medically necessary to permit or facilitate the patient's departure from the hospital, and a limited supply is required until the patient can obtain a continuing supply, the limited supply of the drug or biological is covered as an inpatient hospital service.

SUPPLIES, APPLIANCES, AND EQUIPMENT

Supplies, appliances, and equipment, which are ordinarily furnished by the hospital for the care and treatment of the beneficiary solely during the inpatient hospital stay, are covered inpatient hospital services. Under certain circumstances, supplies, appliances, and equipment used during the beneficiary's inpatient stay are covered under the supplies, appliances and equipment leave the hospital with the patient upon discharge.

These are circumstances in which it would be unreasonable or impossible from a medical standpoint to limit the patient's use of the item to the periods during which the individual is an inpatient.

Examples of items covered under this rule are:

- Items permanently installed in or attached to the patient's body while an inpatient, such as cardiac valves, cardiac pacemakers, and artificial limbs; and
- Items which are temporarily installed in or attached to the patient's body while an inpatient, and which are also necessary to permit or facilitate the patient's release from the hospital, such as tracheotomy or drainage tubes.

Hospital "admission packs" containing primarily toilet articles, such as soap, toothbrushes, toothpaste, and combs, are covered if routinely furnished by the hospital to all its inpatients. If not routinely furnished to all patients, the packs are not covered.

In that situation, the hospital may charge beneficiaries for the pack, but only if they request it with knowledge of what they are requesting and what the charge to them will be. Supplies, appliances, and equipment furnished to an inpatient for use only outside the hospital are not, in general, covered as inpatient hospital services. However, a temporary or disposable item, which is medically necessary to permit or facilitate the patient's departure from the hospital and is required until the patient can obtain a continuing supply, is covered as an inpatient hospital service.

OTHER DIAGNOSTIC OR THERAPEUTIC ITEMS OR SERVICES

Other diagnostic or therapeutic items or services ordinarily furnished inpatients by the hospital or by others under arrangements made by the hospital are covered. This category of covered services encompasses items and services not otherwise specifically listed as covered inpatient hospital services. Such services to hospital inpatients may be covered even when furnished off the hospital premises. For example, diagnostic or therapeutic services of an audiologist off the hospital premises are covered if billed for by the hospital under arrangements, if the services are furnished at a speech and hearing center, and if the audiologist meets the qualifications for an audiologist:

- Is licensed if applicable by the State in which practicing; and
- Is eligible for a certification of clinical competence in audiology granted by the American Speech and Hearing Association; or
- Meets the education requirements for certification and is in the process of accumulating the supervised experience required for certification.

Therapeutic Items

Therapeutic items, which are covered when ordinarily furnished by the hospital to its inpatients, or when ordinarily furnished to hospital inpatients by others under arrangements with them made by the hospital, include but are not limited to the following:

- Surgical dressings, and splints, casts, and other devices used for the reduction of fractures and dislocations;
- Prosthetic devices (other than dental) which replace all or part of an internal body organ (including contiguous tissue) or replace all or part of the function of a permanently inoperative or malfunctioning internal body organ; and
- Leg, arm, back, and neck braces, trusses, and artificial legs, arms, and eyes.

With respect to items that leave the hospital with the patient upon discharge, such as splints or casts, the rules for determining whether the item is covered are the same as the rules set forth above for supplies, appliances, and equipment.

Diagnostic Services of Psychologists and Physical Therapists

When a psychologist or physical therapist is a salaried member of the staff of a hospital, their diagnostic or therapeutic services to inpatients of that hospital are covered.

Independent Clinical Laboratory Under Arrangements With the Hospital

Diagnostic services furnished to an inpatient by an independent clinical laboratory under arrangements with the hospital are reimbursable under hospital insurance provided the lab is certified by CLIA to perform the services. An independent laboratory is one which is independent both of an attending or consulting physician's office and also independent of any hospital which meets at least the requirements to qualify as an emergency hospital (*e.g.*, maintains clinical records, has a utilization review plan, meets the health and safety requirements found necessary by the Secretary of Health and Human Services).

A consulting physician is one whose services include history taking, examination of the patient and, in each case, furnishing to the attending physician an opinion regarding diagnosis or treatment. A physician providing clinical laboratory services for patients of other physicians is not considered to be a consulting physician.

A laboratory operated by or under the supervision of a hospital (or the organized medical staff of the hospital) that does not meet at least the definition of an emergency hospital is considered to be an independent laboratory. However, a laboratory serving hospital patients and operated on the premises of a hospital that meets the definition of an emergency hospital is presumed to be subject to the supervision of the hospital or its organized medical staff and is not an independent laboratory.

A laboratory that a physician or group of physicians maintains for performing diagnostic tests in connection with their own or the group practice is also not considered to be an independent laboratory. An out-of-hospital laboratory is ordinarily presumed to be independent unless there is written evidence establishing that it is operated by or under the supervision of a hospital that meets at least the definition of an emergency hospital or of the organized medical staff of such a hospital.

Refer to "The Conditions of Participation for Hospitals" found at 42 CFR 482 and below for a description of independent lab approval requirements when the hospital is participating. Where a laboratory operated on hospital premises is claimed to be independent or where an out-of-hospital facility is designated as a hospital laboratory, the CMS regional office makes the determination concerning the laboratory's status.

A clinical laboratory is a laboratory where microbiological, serological, chemical, hematological, radiobioassay, cytological, immunohematological, or pathological examinations are performed on materials derived from the human body, to provide information for the diagnosis, prevention, or treatment of a disease or assessment of a medical condition. The "Conditions of Participation for Hospitals (HIRM-1)" call for independent clinical laboratory services furnished under arrangements made by a hospital to be furnished only by a laboratory meeting the specified conditions for coverage under the programme.

These require that:

- Where State or applicable local law provides for licensing of independent clinical laboratories, the laboratory is either licensed under law or is approved as meeting the requirements for licensing by the State or local agency responsible for licensing laboratories; and
- Such laboratories also meet the health and safety requirements prescribed by the Secretary of Health and Human Services..

Where independent laboratory services are provided to patients of a participating hospital under arrangements with the hospital, the law does not require as a condition of payment in an individual case that the independent laboratory be approved under the programme. In processing individual claims, the intermediary, therefore, need not verify that the services were obtained from an approved laboratory.

The intermediary should make payment for laboratory services although it may know that the laboratory from which the hospital has obtained the service is not approved under the programme. However, it should promptly refer this information to the appropriate regional office for review of the determination of the hospital's compliance with the conditions of participation and for whatever action the regional office deems appropriate.

The above policy applies to PPS exempt hospitals. Note that under PPS, there is no separate payment for lab services furnished to inpatients.

Laboratory of Another Participating Hospital

Diagnostic services furnished a hospital inpatient under arrangements with the laboratory of another participating hospital are reimbursable on a cost basis to the hospital obtaining the services if the hospital is PPS exempt.

If the hospital is not exempt, there is not separate payment for lab services furnished to inpatients:

- *NOTE:* Where a PPS exempt hospital obtains diagnostic laboratory services for inpatients under arrangements described in §§50.3 and 50.4 the cost to the hospital obtaining the services would be the reasonable charge for the laboratory's service.

SERVICES OF INTERNS OR RESIDENTS-IN-TRAINING

Hospital insurance covers the reasonable cost of the services of medical or osteopathic interns or residents in training under a teaching programme approved by the appropriate approving body. In the case of services of interns or residents-in-training in the field of dentistry in a hospital or osteopathic hospital, the teaching programme must have the approval of the Council on Dental Education of the American Dental Association.

The services of interns and residents-in-training in the field of podiatry who are in a residency programme approved by the Council on Podiatric Medical Education of the American Podiatric Medical Association are covered on the same basis as the services of other interns and residents in other approved residency programmes.

INPATIENT SERVICES IN CONNECTION WITH DENTAL SERVICES

When a patient is hospitalized for a dental procedure and the dentist's service is covered, the inpatient hospital services furnished. For example, both the professional services of the dentist and the inpatient hospital expenses are covered when the dentist reduces a jaw fracture of an inpatient at a participating hospital.

In addition, hospital inpatient services, which are necessary because of the patient's underlying medical condition and clinical status or the severity of a non-covered dental procedure, are covered.

When the hospital services are covered, all ancillary services such as x-rays, administration of anesthesia, use of the operating room, etc., are covered. Regardless of whether the inpatient hospital services are covered, the medical services of physicians furnished in connection with non-covered dental services are not covered.

The services of an anesthesiologist, radiologist, or pathologist whose services are performed in connection with the care, treatment, filling, removal, or replacement of teeth or structures directly supporting teeth are not covered.

HEALTH CARE ASSOCIATED WITH PREGNANCY

Reasonable and necessary services associated with pregnancy are covered and reimbursable under the Medicare programme. Because pregnancy is a condition sufficiently at variance with the usual state of health, it is appropriate for a pregnant woman to seek medical care. The increased possibility of illness or injury accompanying this condition is well recognized, and medical supervision is required throughout pregnancy and for a brief period beyond. Skilled medical management is appropriate throughout the events of pregnancy, beginning with diagnosis of the condition, continuing through delivery, and ending after the necessary postnatal care.

Similarly, if the pregnancy terminates, whether spontaneously or for therapeutic reasons (*i.e.*, where the life of the mother would be endangered if the fetus were brought to term), the need for skilled medical management and/or medical services is equally as important as in those cases carried to full term. After the infant is delivered, items and services furnished to the infant cannot be covered and reimbursed under the programme on the basis of the mother's eligibility.

TERMINATION OF PREGNANCY

Effective for services furnished on or after October 1, 1998, Medicare will cover abortions procedures in the following situations:

- If the pregnancy is the result of an act or rape or incest; or
- In the case where a woman suffers from a physical disorder, physical injury, or physical illness, including a life-endangering physical condition caused by the pregnancy itself that would, as certified by a physician, place the woman in danger of death unless an abortion is performed.

The "G7" modifier must be used with the following CPT codes in order for these services to be covered when the pregnancy resulted from rape or incest, or the pregnancy is certified by a physician as life threatening to the mother:

- 59840 59841 59850
- 59851 59852 59855
- 59856 59857 59866

TREATMENT FOR INFERTILITY

Effective for services rendered on or after January 15, 1980, reasonable and necessary services associated with treatment for infertility are covered under Medicare. Like pregnancy, infertility is a condition sufficiently at variance with the usual state of health to make it appropriate for a person who normally would be expected to be fertile to seek medical consultation and treatment.

Contractors should coordinate with QIOs to see that utilization guidelines are established for this treatment if inappropriate utilization or abuse is suspected.

4

Laboratory Information Management System

A Laboratory Information Management System (LIMS), sometimes referred to as a Laboratory Information System (LIS) or Laboratory Management System (LMS), is a software-based laboratory and information management system that offers a set of key features that support a modern laboratory's operations. Those key features include — but are not limited to — workflow and data tracking support, flexible architecture, and smart data exchange interfaces, which fully "support its use in regulated environments."The features and uses of a LIMS have evolved over the years from simple sample tracking to an enterprise resource planning tool that manages multiple aspects of laboratory informatics.

The definition of a LIMS is somewhat controversial: LIMSs are dynamic because the modern laboratory's requirements are rapidly evolving and needs often vary significantly from lab to lab. Therefore, a working definition of a LIMS ultimately depends on the interpretation by the individuals or groups involved. Dr. Alan McLelland of the Institute of Biochemistry, Royal Infirmary, Glasgow highlighted this problem in the late 1990s by explaining how a LIMS is perceived by an analyst, a laboratory manager, an information systems manager, and an accountant, "all of them correct, but each of them limited by the users' own perceptions."

Historically the LIMS, LIS, and Process Development Execution System (PDES) have all performed similar functions. Historically the term "LIMS" has tended to be used to reference informatics systems targeted for environmental, research, or commercial analysis such as pharmaceutical or petrochemical work. "LIS" has tended to be used to reference laboratory informatics systems in the forensics and clinical markets, which often required special case management tools. The term "PDES" has generally applied to a wider scope, including, for example, virtual manufacturing techniques, while not necessarily integrating with laboratory equipment.

In recent times LIMS functionality has spread even farther beyond its original purpose of sample management. Assay data management, data mining, data analysis, and electronic laboratory notebook (ELN) integration are all features that have been added to many LIMS, enabling the realization of translational medicine completely within a single software solution. Additionally, the distinction between a LIMS and a LIS has blurred, as many LIMS now also fully support comprehensive case-centric clinical data.

History

Up until the late 1970s, the management of laboratory samples and the associated analysis and reporting were time-consuming manual processes often riddled with transcription errors. This gave some organizations impetus to streamline the collection of data and how it was reported. Custom in-house solutions were developed by a few individual laboratories, while some enterprising entities at the same time sought to develop a more commercial reporting solution in the form of special instrument-based systems.

In 1982 the first generation of LIMS was introduced in the form of a single centralized minicomputer, which offered laboratories the first opportunity to utilize automated reporting tools. As the interest in these early LIMS grew, industry leaders like Gerst Gibbon of the Federal Energy Technology Centre in Pittsburgh began planting the seeds through LIMS-related conferences.

By 1988 the second-generation commercial offerings were tapping into relational databases to expand LIMS into more application-specific territory, and International LIMS Conferences were in full swing. As personal computers became more powerful and prominent, a third generation of LIMS emerged in the early 1990s. These new LIMS took advantage of the developing client/server architecture, allowing laboratories to implement better data processing and exchanges.

By 1995 the client/server tools had developed to the point of allowing processing of data anywhere on the network. Web-enabled LIMS were introduced the following year, enabling researchers to extend operations outside the confines of the laboratory. From 1996 to 2002 additional functionality was included in LIMS, from wireless networking capabilities and georeferencing of samples, to the adoption of XML standards and the development of Internet purchasing.

As of 2012, some LIMS have added additional characteristics that continue to shape how a LIMS is defined. Examples include the addition of clinical functionality, electronic laboratory notebook (ELN) functionality, as well a rise in the software as a service (SaaS) distribution model.

HEALTH SECTOR REFORM AND DECENTRALIZATION

Ghana's long-term vision for growth and development was captured in the document "'GHANA VISION 2020" which sets the scene for decentralised planning. The district is the main implementation unit that prepares annualised plans for development purposes. The Medium Term Health Strategy and the first 5-Year Programme of Work documents, which are the main policy documents that directed the Health Sector Reform in Ghana, were derived essentially from the document GHANA VISION 2020.

Health sector reform started in Ghana within an environment of instability in the early 1980s at a time when national governance was in disarray, there was a severe economic crisis and human development efforts were at a standstill.

Health sector decentralisation was initiated at a time when decision-making at central level (MOH) was seen to be thwarted by bureaucracy and delays with the result that programme implementation was slow and health care service delivery was inefficient and of low quality.

Also at the peripheral level, decision-making capacity was considered low. The Local Government Act of 1993 envisaged a devolution, whereby the responsibility to manage the district health services would be assigned to the district assembly, the locally elected political authority.

In practice, the decentralisation took rather the form of a delegation from the Ministry of Health to the autonomous Ghana Health Service, formalised by the passage of the Ghana Health Service and Teaching Hospitals Act in 1996. The constitution of the Ghana Health Service (GHS) effectively introduced a provider-purchaser split. The Ministry of Health was to take on the roles of policy setting, regulation and accreditation, while the execution of the health policies, including the service delivery, was to become the responsibility of the GHS.

It should be noted that as a result, the Ghana Health Service falls outside the general public service. Through the process of "Strengthening District Health Systems Initiative", a district health system model fashioned around the District Health Management Team was created with deconcentration of decision-making authority and management responsibility between 1986 and 1990.

District Health Management Teams have been targeted for capacity strengthening through short courses and MPH training since the 1980s and block funding replaced the prior allocation mechanism of line budgeting in 1995.

In the First 5-Year Programme of Work, the policy dealt with the orientation of secondary and tertiary service delivery to support primary health services and with the development and implementation of a programme to train adequate numbers of new health teams to provide and manage the health services.

In response, the general policy direction was to decentralise the personnel management procedures to the regional and district levels including the authority to hire and fire in accordance with the deconcentration from the central level of the GHS to the district and regional level.

The promotion of lower staff cadres was delegated to the regional level together with personnel management and salary administration. The goal of human resource development in the health sector was to produce and retain optimal numbers of appropriately trained health workers, placed and motivated to deliver quality health services in areas where the need is highest. Also contracting of human resources for health and performance-based incentive systems have now been introduced.

It should be noted that the tight financial regime imposed by the World Bank had led to retrenchment in the public service (mainly of the unskilled labour categories and euphemistically called 'redeployment') and a partial recruitment freeze, which was ended only in 1997.

THE LABORATORY ENVIRONMENT

The technological revolution now taking place is having a significant impact on the laboratory information management system (LIMS), since such systems are designed to manage the laboratory data. LIMS are information management systems that connect the analytical instruments in the lab to one or more workstations or personal computers. These instruments—such as chromatographs—are used to collect data. An instrument interface is used to forward the data from the chromatograph to the PC, where the data is organized into meaningful information. This information is further sorted and organized into various report formats based upon the type of report required.

It is odd to realize that fewer than seven years ago these systems were simple character-based solutions with green screens. The introduction of Windows-based systems, combined with the demands for very specific format and reporting requirements, have driven the development of LIMS that incorporate the latest technologies—and product delivery concepts driven by those technologies—in innovative ways. One of those concepts is applications on tap.

Applications on Tap

"Apps on tap" comprise an exciting area that is just emerging. Software solutions can be accessed over the Internet rather than the old way of buying a package off the shelf and installing it on the hard drive or server. Application service providers, or ASPs, are organizations that offer software solutions remotely over the Internet to companies that pay service and transaction fees to access the solution.

The earliest manifestation of apps on tap came about with e-mail and Internet access, such as AOL's initial offering. Now, AOL bundles Internet access, e-mail, shopping, chat rooms, and more into a robust product that's both easy to use and buy. A monthly fee is paid, a user name is issued, and the solution is installed and the user online in minutes.

There are a slew of dot. coms emerging with just about every conceivable take on this concept. For instance, there are organizations that offer supply chain management programs remotely for company purchasers and vendors to enable transactions between buyers and sellers.

SAP, the enterprise resource planning system provider, is now offering a hosted option for their system solutions. Existing customers are buying additional licenses and moving to the hosted environment. The enterprise resource planning solutions SAP offers, however, are only available from certified host partners. They handle all the computers and provide low-level system expertise and upgrades if needed, plus services such as capacity planning.

A new spin on the ASP is the vertical service provider that hosts another organization's applications. Companies such as Portera Systems fall into this category. Portera distributes Oracle's financial, human resources, and purchasing applications online.

There is even a start-up called AppCity that bills itself as an application portal and offers information-based applications for business users and consumers. The site launched with 50 applications in four categories: business, information, lifestyle, and shopping. These applications, however, are more like spreadsheets that let users view or chart information than full-blown Windows applications.

On the LIMS front, this concept was recently addressed by LabVantage Solutions with the introduction of their @LIMS product. @LIMS is a web-based solution that eliminates the need for the user to purchase many of the LIMS components with a thin client, 4MB footprint that operates from a T1 line at LabVantage's offices. Similar in concept to an Internet service provider (ISP), solution, time, and capabilities—including data storage, support, maintenance, upgrades, and training—are purchased on a monthly basis.

It is designed for small labs of five to 10 people. This is a concept along the lines of Oracle Corporation's premature attempt in the early 1990s to sell a network computer similar to the dumb terminals of the early 1980s. This network computer would dial into a central server that hosted all the applications which could then be accessed for a monthly fee. A pay-as-you-go, drop-it-on-your-credit-card concept similar to the business model used by AOL and other Internet service providers, it was a great idea, but before its time. When Oracle originally proposed that concept in the early 1990s, the Internet's physical infrastructure was not as robust as it is now and the security features not as sophisticated. The market may be ready now. However, one of the problems then, and which still exists, is that the browser interface is not very powerful. It's not yet possible to have all the functionality of a desktop application with just a Web browser and Java. So, the ability to use Windows-like features—such as dragging and dropping an item within a window—appears to be key to full-scale market acceptance of ASP solutions.

The Virtual Desktop

Storage solutions may continue to improve at the desktop level. Certainly there will be vendors who will capitalize on this need by offering ever more robust solutions. There will also be organizations, applications, and requirements that dictate a desktop solution.

Future storage solutions may migrate in greater numbers to the server, however. This certainly seems likely as business processes will no doubt continue to migrate toward a Web-centric approach, with data, information, and applications stored somewhere other than on the physical desktop. Wireless functionality will help in this arena. For instance, Analytical Automation Specialists offers a Field Data Entry Terminal that allows remote access to the LIMS via a PCMCIA (Personal Computer Memory card International Association) modem. This small Windows palmtop provides a global positioning satellite (GPS) system for georeferencing and is particularly appropriate for environmental and petrochemical applications. Samples can be logged in from the field and cross-referenced based on absolute latitude and longitude at ±10 feet [3 m].

If a laptop or palmtop can access or deliver information from any place where satellite transmissions are possible, then it makes more sense to host data and applications on a server than it does to keep it on an inaccessible desktop. This is a productivity issue. Does this indicate that the virtual desktop is the next revolution that will take place in the office? If office applications migrate to the server, where LIMS information is usually kept, then it makes sense to integrate the two ever more tightly.

Will we finally realize the paperless office? Indeed, the paperless office is getting closer. The FDA's 21 CFR Part 11 rule for electronic records and signatures has defined the standard that eliminates the need for a paper trail when there is an electronic one. But the concept of the paperless office relies upon a robust computer system.

One more point to consider: More and more businesses consider corporate knowledge more important than the product they sell. It's what you know that counts. Thus what differentiates an organization from its competitors may be what it has learned about producing the product as much as the actual product itself. Knowledge management is thus being touted as the next arena for competitive differentiation.

Knowledge management is defined as the processes that are applied to the acquisition, storage, and dissemination of an organization's knowledge assets. It is not an IS (information systems) activity, but falls within the IT (information technology) infrastructure, hence an organization's information management solutions —such as the LIMS— are fundamental components of the knowledge management strategy. Simply put, knowledge management represents the processes required to bring the right information to the right people at the right time. It is anticipated that knowledge management requirements will be one of the driving forces behind the next-generation LIMS.

The Next-Generation LIMS and the Virtual Lab

There are so many different potential realities, so many converging technologies and capabilities that can have a dramatic impact on the next-generation LIMS. E-commerce. Internet marketplaces. Apps on tap. Web browser access. Bandwidth control. Storage technology. Faster, better, cheaper chips. Knowledge management.

The above activity seems comparable to timelines of the earth's history where mankind occupies just the last few seconds in the total life of the planet. Just a blip. LIMS are still in an adolescent phase, so the turn of the century has little meaning as a milestone. The first 20 years of the automated lab are past. The next 20 years should prove very interesting indeed, now that telecommunications plays such a significant role in data management. We'll be doing things in the lab in 2020 that are not even imaginable today. And bragging about how tough we had it in the old days!

There's an interesting comparison to be made between the 40-year stretch that began in the 1880s and the current one that began in the 1980s. During the first 40-year span, industrialized society moved from gas lamps to electric ones, from horse and buggy to automobile, from clipper ships to airplanes. What amazing changes these must have been! Those changes appear so simple compared to the complexity of the situation in which we find ourselves today.

Of course, it was not easy to create an infrastructure for a regional, let alone national, electrical system. Nor was it easy to define and enforce traffic laws that brought some sanity to driving on the roads. But, today, we're faced with legacy infrastructures that must be managed so that new systems and capabilities can be overlaid over existing, often obsolete, systems without impacting business negatively.

Where we have been depends so much on where we are going. The seeds have been sown and some are beginning to sprout. Web-based LIMS are now common. Electronic lab notebooks have become ubiquitous in the lab. LabVantage Solutions has already introduced the first LIMS packaged as an app on tap. NuGenesis Technologies, on the other hand, is attempting to create a new market arena for their Scientific Data Management

System product, which allows users to archive and unify scientific information generated in the laboratory to a common database. From this central repository, information can be viewed, mapped, mined, analyzed, organized, shared, and reused.

This solution is quite obviously the marriage of laboratory information requirements with enterprise-management information requirements. Solutions such as this, which leverage the best of a range of technologies, are what drive the convergence of those technologies. Is this the next-generation LIMS? It has many of the components of a knowledge management system. Will the virtual lab ever exist? You can probably count on it. What will it look like? No doubt both familiar and strange.

It is important to remember that LIMS are being squeezed between competing applications. Will they soon be swallowed by instrument-centric solutions or enterprise-centric ones? These scenarios are both highly likely and somewhat improbable, and whether or not either occurs depends on the upcoming unpredictable twists of technology that will drive the market down a given path.

Technology and Operations

The LIMS is an evolving concept, with new features and functionality being added often. As laboratory demands change and technological progress continues, the functions of a LIMS will likely also change. Despite these changes, a LIMS tends to have a base set of functionality that defines it. That functionality can roughly be divided into five laboratory processing phases,

With numerous software functions falling under each:

- The reception and log in of a sample and its associated customer data.
- The assignment, scheduling, and tracking of the sample and the associated analytical workload.
- The processing and quality control associated with the sample and the utilized equipment and inventory.
- The storage of data associated with the sample analysis.
- The inspection, approval, and compilation of the sample data for reporting and/or further analysis.

There are several pieces of core functionality associated with these laboratory processing phases that tend to appear in most LIMS:

Sample Management

The core function of LIMS has traditionally been the management of samples. This typically is initiated when a sample is received in the laboratory, at which point the sample will be registered in the LIMS. Some LIMS will allow the customer to place an "order" for a sample directly to the LIMS at which point the sample is generated in an "unreceived" state. The processing could then include a step where the sample container is registered and sent to the customer for the sample to be taken and then returned to the lab. The registration process may involve accessioning the sample and producing barcodes to affix to the sample container.

Various other parameters such as clinical or phenotypic information corresponding with the sample are also often recorded. The LIMS then tracks chain of custody as well as sample location. Location tracking usually involves assigning the sample to a particular freezer location, often down to the granular level of shelf, rack, box, row, and column. Other event tracking such as freeze and thaw cycles that a sample undergoes in the laboratory may be required.

Modern LIMS have implemented extensive configurability, as each laboratory's needs for tracking additional data points can vary widely. LIMS vendors cannot typically make assumptions about what these data tracking needs are, and therefore vendors must create LIMS that are adaptable to individual environments. LIMS users may also have regulatory concerns to comply with such as CLIA, HIPAA, GLP, and FDA specifications, affecting certain aspects of sample management in a LIMS solution. One key to compliance with many of these standards is audit logging of all changes to LIMS data, and in some cases a full electronic signature system is required for rigorous tracking of field-level changes to LIMS data.

Instrument and Application Integration

Modern LIMS offer an increasing amount of integration with laboratory instruments and applications. A LIMS may create control files that are "fed" into the instrument and direct its operation on some physical item such as a sample tube or sample plate. The LIMS may then import instrument results files to extract data for quality control assessment of the operation on the sample. Access to the instrument data can sometimes be regulated based on chain of custody assignments or other security features if need be.

Modern LIMS products now also allow for the import and management of raw assay data results. Modern targeted assays such as qPCR and deepsequencing can produce tens of thousands of data points per sample. Furthermore, in the case of drug and diagnostic development as many as 12 or more assays may be run for each sample. In order to track this data, a LIMS solution needs to be adaptable to many different assay formats at both the data layer and import creation layer, while maintaining a high level of overall performance. Some LIMS products address this by simply attaching assay data as BLOBs to samples, but this limits the utility of that data in data mining and downstream analysis.

Electronic Data Exchange

The exponentially growing volume of data created in laboratories, coupled with increased business demands and focus on profitability, have pushed LIMS vendors to increase attention to how their LIMS handles electronic data exchanges. Attention must be paid to how an instrument's input and output data is managed, how remote sample collection data is imported and exported, and how mobile technology integrates with the LIMS. The successful transfer of data files in Microsoft Excel and other formats, as well as the import and export of data to Oracle, SQL, and Microsoft Access databases is a pivotal aspect of the modern LIMS. In fact, the transition "from proprietary databases to standardized database management systems such as Oracle ... and SQL" has arguably had one of the biggest impacts on how data is managed and exchanged in laboratories.

Additional Functions

Aside from the key functions of sample management, instrument and application integration, and electronic data exchange, there are numerous additional operations that can be managed in a LIMS.

This includes but is not limited to:

- Audit management: fully track and maintain an audit trail.
- Barcode handling: assign one or more data points to a barcode format; read and extract information from a barcode.
- Chain of custody: assign roles and groups that dictate access to specific data records and who is managing them
- Compliance: follow regulatory standards that affect the laboratory.
- Customer relationship management: handle the demographic information and communications for associated clients.

- Document management: process and convert data to certain formats; manage how documents are distributed and accessed.
- Instrument calibration and maintenance: schedule important maintenance and calibration of lab instruments and keep detailed records of such activities.
- Inventory and equipment management: measure and record inventories of vital supplies and laboratory equipment.
- Manual and electronic data entry: provide fast and reliable interfaces for data to be entered by a human or electronic component.
- Method management: provide one location for all laboratory process and procedure (P&P) and methodology to be housed and managed as well as connecting each sample handling step with current instructions for performing the operation.
- Personnel and workload management: organize work schedules, workload assignments, employee demographic information, training, and financial information.
- Quality assurance and control: gauge and control sample quality, data entry standards, and workflow.
- Reports: create and schedule reports in a specific format; schedule and distribute reports to designated parties.
- Time tracking: calculate and maintain processing and handling times on chemical reactions, workflows, and more.
- Traceability: show audit trail and/or chain of custody of a sample.
- Workflows: track a sample, a batch of samples, or a "lot" of batches through its lifecycle.

Client-Side Options

A LIMS has utilized many architectures and distribution models over the years. As technology has changed, how a LIMS is installed, managed, and utilized has also changed with it. The following represents architectures which have been utilized at one point or another:

Thick-Client

A thick-client LIMS is a more traditional client/server architecture, with some of the system residing on the computer or workstation of the user (the client) and the rest on the server. The LIMS software is installed on the client computer, which does all of the data processing. Later it passes information to the server, which has the primary purpose of data storage. Most changes, upgrades, and other modifications will happen on the client side. This was one of the first architectures implemented into a LIMS, having the advantage of providing higher processing speeds (because processing is done on the client and not the server) and slightly more security (as access to the server data is limited only to those with client software).

Additionally, thick-client systems have also provided more interactivity and customization, though often at a greater learning curve. The disadvantages of client-side LIMS include the need for more robust client computers and more time-consuming upgrades, as well as a lack of base functionality through a web browser. The thick-client LIMS can become web-enabled through an add-on component.

Thin-Client

A thin-client LIMS is a more modern architecture which offers full application functionality accessed through a device's web browser. The actual LIMS software resides on a server (host) which feeds and processes information without saving it to the user's hard disk. Any necessary changes, upgrades, and other modifications are handled by the entity hosting the server-side LIMS software, meaning all end-users see all changes made. To this end, a true thin-client LIMS will leave no "footprint" on the client's computer, and only the integrity of the web browser need be maintained by the user.

The advantages of this system include significantly lower cost of ownership and fewer network and client-side maintenance expenses. However, this architecture has the disadvantage of requiring real-time server access, a need for increased network throughput, and slightly less functionality. A sort of hybrid architecture that incorporates the features of thin-client browser usage with a thick client installation exists in the form of a web-based LIMS.

Some LIMS vendors are beginning to rent hosted, thin-client solutions as "software as a service" (SaaS). These solutions tend to be less configurable than on premise solutions and are therefore considered for less demanding implementations such as laboratories with few users and limited sample processing volumes.

Another implementation of the thin client architecture is the maintenance, warranty, and support (MSW) agreement. Pricing levels are typically based on a percentage of the license fee, with a standard level of service for 10 concurrent users being approximately 10 hours of support and additional customer service, at a roughly $200 per hour rate. Though some may choose to opt out of an MSW after the first year, it's often more economical to continue the plan in order to receive updates to the LIMS, giving it a longer life span in the laboratory.

Web-Enabled

A web-enabled LIMS architecture is essentially a thick-client architecture with an added web browser component. In this setup, the client-side software has additional functionality that allows users to interface with the software through their device's browser. This functionality is typically limited only to certain functions of the web client. The primary advantage of a web-enabled LIMS is the end-user can access data both on the client side and the server side of the configuration. As in a thick-client architecture, updates in the software must be propagated to every client machine. However, the added disadvantages of requiring always-on access to the host server and the need for cross-platform functionality mean that additional overhead costs may arise.

Web-Based

Arguably one of the most confusing architectures, web-based LIMS architecture is a hybrid of the thick- and thin-client architectures. While much of the client-side work is done through a web browser, the LIMS also requires the additional support of Microsoft's .NET Framework technology installed on the client device. The end result is a process that is apparent to the end-user through the Microsoft-compatible web browser, but perhaps not so apparent as it runs thick-client-like processing in the background. In this case, web-based architecture has the advantage of providing more functionality through a more friendly web interface. The disadvantages of this setup are more sunk costs in system administration and support for Internet Explorer and .NET technologies, and reduced functionality on mobile platforms.

Configurability

LIMS implementations are notorious for often being lengthy and costly. This is due in part to the diversity of requirements within each lab, but also to the inflexible nature of LIMS products for adapting to these widely varying requirements. Newer LIMS solutions are beginning to emerge that take advantage of modern techniques in software design that are inherently more configurable and adaptable — particularly at the data layer — than prior solutions. This means not only that implementations are much faster, but also that the costs are lower and the risk of obsolescence is minimized.

MEDICAL LABORATORY

A medical laboratory or clinical laboratory is a laboratory where tests are done on clinical specimens in order to get information about the health of a patient as pertaining to the diagnosis, treatment, and prevention of disease.

Departments

Laboratory medicine is generally divided into four sections, and each of which is further divided into a number of units. These four sections are:

- Anatomic Pathology: units are included here, namely histopathology, cytopathology, and electron microscopy. Academically, each unit is studied alone in one course. Other courses pertaining to this section include anatomy, physiology, histology, pathology, and pathophysiology.
- Clinical Microbiology: This is the largest section in laboratory medicine; as it encompasses five different sciences (units). These include bacteriology, virology, parasitology, immunology, and mycology.
- Clinical Biochemistry: Units under this busy section are instrumental analysis, enzymology, toxicology and endocrinology.
- Hematology: This busy, section consists of three units, which are coagulation and blood bank and hematology.

Genetics is also studied along with a subspecialty known as cytogenetics. Distribution of clinical laboratories in health institutions varies greatly from one place to another. Take for example microbiology, some health facilities have a single laboratory for microbiology, while others have a separate lab for each unit, with nothing called a "microbiology" lab. Here's a detailed breakdown of the responsibilities of each unit:

- Microbiology receives almost any clinical specimen, including swabs, feces, urine, blood, sputum, cerebrospinal fluid, synovial fluid, as well as possible infected tissue. The work here is mainly concerned with cultures, to look for suspected pathogens which, if found, are further identified based on biochemical tests. Also, sensitivity testing is carried out to determine whether the pathogen is sensitive or resistant to a suggested medicine. Results are reported with the identified organism(s) and the type and amount of drug(s) that should be prescribed for the patient.

- Parasitology is a microbiology unit that investigates parasites. The most frequently encountered specimen here is faeces. However, blood, urine, sputum, and other samples may also contain parasites.
- Virology is concerned with identification of viruses in specimens such as blood, urine, and cerebrospinal fluid.
- Hematology works with whole blood to do full blood counts, and blood films as well as many other specialised tests.
- Coagulation requires citrated blood samples to analyze blood clotting times and coagulation factors.
- Clinical Biochemistry usually receives serum or plasma. They test the serum for chemicals present in blood. These include a wide array of substances, such as lipids, blood sugar, enzymes, and hormones.
- Toxicology mainly tests for pharmaceutical and recreational drugs. Urine and blood samples are submitted to this lab.
- Immunology/Serology uses the concept of antigen-antibody interaction as a diagnostic tool. Compatibility of transplanted organs is also determined.
- Immunohaematology, or Blood bank determines blood groups, and performs compatibility testing on blood donors and recipients. It also prepares blood components, derivatives, and products for transfusion.
- Urinalysis tests urine for many analytes. Some health care providers have a urinalysis laboratory, while others don't. Instead, each component of the urinalysis is performed at the corresponding unit. If measuring urine chemicals is required, the specimen is processed in the clinical biochemistry lab, but if cell studies are indicated, the specimen should be submitted to the cytopathology lab, and so on.
- Histopathology processes solid tissue removed from the body (biopsies) for evaluation at the microscopic level.
- Cytopathology examines smears of cells from all over the body (such as from the cervix) for evidence of inflammation, cancer, and other conditions.

- Electron microscopy prepares specimens and takes micrographs of very fine details by means of TEM and SEM.
- Genetics mainly performs DNA analysis.
- Cytogenetics involves using blood and other cells to get a karyotype. This can be helpful in prenatal diagnosis (e.g. Down's syndrome) as well as in cancer (some cancers have abnormal chromosomes).
- Surgical pathology examines organs, limbs, tumors, fetuses, and other tissues biopsied in surgery such as breast mastectomys.

Medical Laboratory Staff

The following is the hierarchy of the clinical laboratory staff from highest authority to lowest:

- Medical Director
- Pathologist, Clinical Biologist, Microbiologist, Biochemist,
- Resident in Pathology or Clinical Biology
- Pathologist Assistant, Microbiologist Assistant, Medical Biochemist Assistant,
- Laboratory Manager,
- Department Supervisor,
- Chief/Lead Technologist,
- Cytotechnologist, Medical Laboratory Scientist, Histotechnologist,
- Medical Laboratory Technician, Histotechnician
- Medical Laboratory Assistant (Lab Aide),
- Phlebotomist,
- Transcriptionist,
- Specimen processor, Secretary).

Some of these titles don't exist in some countries. Sometimes technologists and technicians do the same work. In France, clinical biologists may also be Medical director and laboratory manager.

SOCIAL AND LEGAL ASPECTS OF HEALTH CARE MANAGEMENT

The modern face of medicine reflects a prodigious and growing range of treatment options. Paralleling this growth, society is witnessing an expanding acceptance of respect for patient autonomy in healthcare decision-making. While acknowledging that active patient involvement in medical management can lead to a more successful outcome, physicians can become frustrated when their advice is ignored or rejected by patients. This dynamic has created both a partnership and tension in the doctor-patient relationship. In England and Scotland, a body of law has developed which has begun to sort out the complex issues that can arise when patients, families and physicians disagree.

Medico- Legal Aspects of the Usage of Electronic Health Record

In the recent years, healthcare organizations are showing an increased rate of acquisition of computer technologies and their spending rates shows an upward tendency placing the industry as one to the major consumers of ICT products and services. Frost & Sullivan estimates the Health Information Technology market (by revenue) in 2008, in APAC (Southeast Asia, China, Japan and Australia) was close to USD5.04 billion with an annual growth rate (CAGR) of 11.8 percent from 2005-2008. Although the APAC HIT market represents currently only 2.1 percent of the total healthcare market, it is very likely that the figure could double if not triple that in the next 10 years.

Dr. Pawel Suwinsk, senior consultant at Frost & Sullivan says, 'The HIT is here to stay with even more ubiquitous presence in all aspects of healthcare delivery systems. Moreover, it will be the main factor and driver in the transformation of healthcare industry towards translation care by providing common collaboration platform for information processing and exchange between related sciences and industries.'

He further elaborates, " 50 percent of the medical practice activities can be controlled. The remaining 50 percent depends solely on human judgment and cognitive functions that when unfavourable conditions are present could lead to substandard care. The implementation of HIT can improve the quality of care by providing better control (up to 80 percent). However, while decreasing the legal exposure of traditional medical practice it introduces legal implications related to the usage of HIT." The following are some of the medico-legal aspects of the usage of healthcare IT solutions including electronic medical records.

Medical liability which is also entitled as medical negligence or medical malpractice is a special component of tort law which governs the professional relationship between physicians and their patients. It is concerned about the duties of care expected between physicians and their patients in delivering health care. It is said that the duty of a physician to his or her patients is to practice medicine which meets or exceeds the standard of care.

If the hospital or healthcare delivery organizations violate standard of care (through inadequate oversight of its staff physicians) by allowing EHR or other technology of its choice to be used in such a way to harm patients, it might become the subject of corporate negligence action. The case of Vicarious liability occurs when there is a design or other type of flaw in any of the technologies including electronic health record or computerized physician order entry that causes harm to patients even though the physicians or other caregivers who uses that committed no negligence.

The unauthorized access to patient's private information results in the privacy violation. User negligence, misdirected information flow or intentional security breach by a third party etc..could be some of the reasons for this information leakage. Security breached is recognized as unauthorized sharing of patient's private information. Inappropriate disclosure can happen in clinical setting when multiple copies of Electronic Health Record (EHR) persist even after destruction of original file is being accessed by unauthorized personnel.

Medical liability actions may also arise from acts of commission which breach the standard of care and result in injury and damages to patients.

Physicians could also find themselves in trouble by failing to use diagnostic and treatment modalities suggested by the embedded best practice guidelines in certain types of electronic health records. Here there could be an act of omission contributing to patient injury.

Some of the preventative measures suggested in the course of medical liability are the selection of appropriate healthcare information system, proper training of staff to ensure efficient use of system, documenting all information with justification (whether or not care provided), and preventing any further alteration to this records without proper documentation etc..

MEDICAL ETHICS

Medical ethics is primarily a field of applied ethics, the study of moral values and judgments as they apply to medicine. As a scholarly discipline, medical ethics encompasses its practical application in clinical settings as well as work on its history, philosophy, theology, and sociology.

Medical ethics tends to be understood narrowly as an applied professional ethics, whereas bioethics appears to have worked more expansive concerns, touching upon the philosophy of science and issues of biotechnology. Still, the two fields often overlap and the distinction is more a matter of style than professional consensus. Medical ethics shares many principles with other branches of healthcare ethics, such as nursing ethics.

History

Historically, Western medical ethics may be traced to guidelines on the duty of physicians in antiquity, such as the Hippocratic Oath, and early rabbinic and Christian teachings. In the medieval and early modern period, the field is indebted to Muslim physicians such as Ishaq bin Ali Rahawi (who wrote the *Conduct of a Physician*, the first book dedicated to medical ethics) and Muhammad ibn Zakariya ar-Razi (known as Rhazes in the West), Jewish thinkers such as Maimonides, Roman Catholic scholastic thinkers such as Thomas Aquinas, and the case-oriented analysis (casuistry) of Catholic moral theology. These intellectual traditions continue in Catholic, Islamic and Jewish medical ethics.

By the 18th and 19th centuries, medical ethics emerged as a more self-conscious discourse. For instance, authors such as Thomas Percival wrote about "medical jurisprudence" and reportedly coined the phrase "medical ethics." Percival's guidelines related to physician consultations have been criticized as being excessively protective of the home physician's reputation. Jeffrey Berlant is one such critic who considers Percival's codes of physician consultations as being an early example of the anti-competitive, "guild"-like nature of the physician community. In 1847, the American Medical Association adopted its first code of ethics, with this being based in large part upon Percival's work. While the secularized field borrowed largely from Catholic medical ethics, in the 20th century a distinctively liberal Protestant approach was articulated by thinkers such as Joseph Fletcher. In the 1960s and 1970s, building upon liberal theory and procedural justice, much of the discourse of medical ethics went through a dramatic shift and largely reconfigured itself into bioethics.

Since the 1970s, the growing influence of ethics in contemporary medicine can be seen in the increasing use of Institutional Review Boards to evaluate experiments on human subjects, the establishment of hospital ethics committees, the expansion of the role of clinician ethicists, and the integration of ethics into many medical school curricula.

Values in Medical Ethics

Six of the values that commonly apply to medical ethics discussions are:

- Autonomy - the patient has the right to refuse or choose their treatment.
- Beneficence - a practitioner should act in the best interest of the patient.
- Non-maleficence - "first, do no harm".
- Justice - concerns the distribution of scarce health resources, and the decision of who gets what treatment (fairness and equality).
- Dignity - the patient (and the person treating the patient) have the right to dignity.
- Truthfulness and honesty - the concept of informed consent has increased in importance since the historical events of the Doctors' Trial of the Nuremberg trials and Tuskegee Syphilis Study.

Values such as these do not give answers as to how to handle a particular situation, but provide a useful framework for understanding conflicts. When moral values are in conflict, the result may be an ethical dilemma or crisis. Sometimes, no good solution to a dilemma in medical ethics exists, and occasionally, the values of the medical community (i.e., the hospital and its staff) conflict with the values of the individual patient, family, or larger non-medical community.

Conflicts can also arise between health care providers, or among family members. Some argue for example, that the principles of autonomy and beneficence clash when patients refuse blood transfusions, considering them life-saving; and truth-telling was not emphasized to a large extent before the HIV era.

Autonomy

The principle of autonomy recognizes the rights of individuals to self determination. This is rooted in society's respect for individuals' ability to make informed decisions about personal matters. Autonomy has become more important as social values have shifted to define medical quality in terms of outcomes that are important to the patient rather than medical professionals. The increasing importance of autonomy can be seen as a social reaction to a "paternalistic" tradition within healthcare. Some have questioned whether the backlash against historically excessive paternalism in favour of patient autonomy has inhibited the proper use of soft paternalism to the detriment of outcomes for some patients. Respect for autonomy is the basis for informed consent and advance directives.

Autonomy is a general indicator of health. Many diseases are characterised by loss of autonomy, in various manners. This makes autonomy an indicator for both personal well-being, and for the well-being of the profession. This has implications for the consideration of medical ethics: "is the aim of health care to do good, and benefit from it?"; or "is the aim of health care to do good to others, and have them, and society, benefit from this?". (Ethics - by definition - tries to find a beneficial balance between the activities of the individual and its effects on a collective.)

By considering Autonomy as a gauge parameter for (self) health care, the medical and ethical perspective both benefit from the implied reference to Health.

Beneficence

The term beneficence refers to actions that promote the wellbeing of others. In the medical context, this means taking actions that serve the best interests of patients. However, uncertainty surrounds the precise definition of which practices do in fact help patients. James Childress and Tom Beauchamp in *Principle of Biomedical Ethics* (1978) identify beneficence as one of the core values of health care ethics. Some scholars, such as Edmund Pellegrino, argue that beneficence is the *only* fundamental principle of medical ethics. They argue that healing should be the sole purpose of medicine, and that endeavors like cosmetic surgery, contraception and euthanasia fall beyond its purview.

Non-Maleficence

The concept of non-maleficence is embodied by the phrase, "first, do no harm," or the Latin, *primum non nocere*. Many consider that should be the main or primary consideration (hence *primum*): that it is more important not to harm your patient, than to do them good. This is partly because enthusiastic practitioners are prone to using treatments that they believe will do good, without first having evaluated them adequately to ensure they do no (or only acceptable levels of) harm. Much harm has been done to patients as a result. It is not only more important to do no harm than to do good; it is also important to *know* how likely it is that your treatment will harm a patient. So a physician should go further than not prescribing medications they know to be harmful - he or she should not prescribe medications (or otherwise treat the patient) unless s/he knows that the treatment is unlikely to be harmful; or at the very least, that patient understands the risks and benefits, and that the likely benefits outweigh the likely risks.

In practice, however, many treatments carry some risk of harm. In some circumstances, e.g. in desperate situations where the outcome without treatment will be grave, risky treatments that stand a high chance of harming the patient will be justified, as the risk of not treating is also very likely to do harm. So the principle of *non-maleficence* is not absolute, and must be balanced against the principle of *beneficence* (doing good).

"Non-maleficence" is defined by its cultural context. Every culture has its own cultural collective definitions of 'good' and 'evil'. Their definitions depend on the degree to which the culture sets its cultural values apart from nature. In some cultures the terms "good" and "evil" are absent: for them these words lack meaning as their experience of nature does not set them apart from nature. Other cultures place the humans in interaction with nature, some even place humans in a position of dominance over nature. The religions are the main means of expression of these considerations. Depending on the cultural consensus conditioning (expressed by its religious, political and legal social system) the legal definition of Non-maleficence differs. Violation of non-maleficence is the subject of medical malpractice litigation. Regulations thereof differ, over time, per nation.

Double Effect

Some interventions undertaken by physicians can create a positive outcome while foreseeably, but unintentionally, doing harm. The combination of these two circumstances is known as the "double effect". A commonly cited, but fallacious, example of this phenomenon is the use of morphine in the dying patient. Such use of morphine can ease the pain and suffering of the patient, while simultaneously hastening the demise of the patient through suppression of the respiratory drive. If correct, this would be an example of the double effect; however, no research evidence supports the claim that appropriately administered opioid drugs depress the respiratory system.

Conflicts between Autonomy and Beneficence/Non-maleficence

Autonomy can come into conflict with Beneficence when patients disagree with recommendations that health care professionals believe are in the patient's best interest. When the patient's interests conflict with the patient's welfare, different societies settle the conflict in a wide range of manners. Western medicine generally defers to the wishes of a mentally competent patient to make his own decisions, even in cases where the medical team believes that he is not acting in his own best interests. However, many other societies prioritize beneficence over autonomy.

Examples include when a patient does not want a treatment because of, for example, religious or cultural views. In the case of euthanasia, the patient, or relatives of a patient, may want to end the life of the patient. Also, the patient may want an unnecessary treatment, as can be the case in hypochondria. A doctor may want to prefer Autonomy because refusal to please the patient's will would harm the doctor-patient relationship. Individuals' capacity for informed decision making may come into question during resolution of conflicts between Autonomy and Beneficence. The role of surrogate medical decision makers is an extension of the principle of autonomy.

Euthanasia

Some American physicians interpret the non-maleficence principle to exclude the practice of euthanasia, though not all concur. Probably the most extreme example in recent history of the violation of the non-maleficence dictum was Dr. Jack Kevorkian, who was convicted of second-degree homicide in Michigan in 1998 after demonstrating active euthanasia on the TV news show, 60 Minutes.

In some countries euthanasia is accepted as standard medical practice. Legal regulations assign this to the medical profession. In such nations, the aim is to alleviate the suffering of patients from diseases known to be incurable by the methods known in that culture. In that sense, the "Primum no Nocere" is based on the realisation that *the inability of the medical expert to offer help, creates a known great and ongoing suffering in the patient.* "Not acting" in those cases is believed to be more damaging than actively relieving the suffering of the patient. Evidently the ability to offer help depends on the limitation of what the practitioner can do. These limitations are characteristic for each different form of healing, and the legal system of the specific culture. The aim to "not do harm" is still the same. It gives the medical practitioner a responsibility to help the patient, in the intentional and active relief of suffering, in those cases where no cure can be offered.

Informed Consent

Informed consent in ethics usually refers to the idea that a person must be fully-informed about and understand the potential benefits and risks of their choice of treatment. An uninformed person is at risk of mistakenly making a choice not reflective of his or her values or wishes. It does not specifically mean the process of obtaining consent, nor the specific legal requirements, which vary from place to place, for capacity to consent. Patients can elect to make their own medical decisions, or can delegate decision-making authority to another party. If the patient is incapacitated, laws around the world designate different processes for obtaining informed consent, typically by having a person appointed by the patient or their next of kin make decisions for them. The value of informed consent is closely related to the values of autonomy and truth telling. A correlate to "informed consent" is the concept of informed refusal.

CONFIDENTIALITY

Confidentiality is commonly applied to conversations between doctors and patients. This concept is commonly known as patient-physician privilege. Legal protections prevent physicians from revealing their discussions with patients, even under oath in court. Confidentiality is mandated in America by HIPAA laws, specifically the Privacy Rule, and various state laws, some more rigorous than HIPAA. However, numerous exceptions to the rules have been carved out over the years. For example, many states require physicians to report gunshot wounds to the police and impaired drivers to the Department of Motor Vehicles. Confidentiality is also challenged in cases involving the diagnosis of a sexually transmitted disease in a patient who refuses to reveal the diagnosis to a spouse, and in the termination of a pregnancy in an underage patient, without the knowledge of the patient's parents. Many states in the U.S. have laws governing parental notification in underage abortion.

Traditionally, medical ethics has viewed the duty of confidentiality as a relatively non-negotiable tenet of medical practice. More recently, critics like Jacob Appel have argued for a more nuanced approach to the duty that acknowledges the need for flexibility in many cases.

Criticisms of Orthodox Medical Ethics

It has been argued that mainstream medical ethics is biased by the assumption of a framework in which individuals are not simply free to contract with one another to provide whatever medical treatment is demanded, subject to the ability to pay. Because a high proportion of medical care is typically provided via the welfare state, and because there are legal restrictions on what treatment may be provided and by whom, an automatic divergence may exist between the wishes of patients and the preferences of medical practitioners and other parties. Tassano has questioned the idea that Beneficence might in some cases have priority over Autonomy. He argues that violations of Autonomy more often reflect the interests of the state or of the supplier group than those of the patient. Routine regulatory professional bodies or the courts of law are valid social recourses.

Importance of Communication

Many so-called "ethical conflicts" in medical ethics are traceable back to a lack of communication. Communication breakdowns between patients and their healthcare team, between family members, or between members of the medical community, can all lead to disagreements and strong feelings. These breakdowns should be remedied, and many apparently insurmountable "ethics" problems can be solved with open lines of communication.

Control and Resolution

To ensure that appropriate ethical values are being applied within hospitals, effective hospital accreditation requires that ethical considerations are taken into account, for example with respect to physician integrity, conflicts of interest, research ethics and organ transplantation ethics.

Guidelines

There are various ethical guidelines. For example, the Declaration of Helsinki is regarded as authoritative in human research ethics. In the United Kingdom, General Medical Council provides clear overall modern guidance in the form of its 'Good Medical Practice' statement. Other organisations, such as the Medical Protection Society and a number of university departments, are often consulted by British doctors regarding issues relating to ethics.

Ethics Committees

Often, simple communication is not enough to resolve a conflict, and a hospital ethics committee must convene to decide a complex matter.

These bodies are composed primarily of health care professionals, but may also include philosophers, lay people, and clergy - indeed, in many parts of the world their presence is considered mandatory in order to provide balance.

With respect to the expected composition of such bodies in the USA, Europe and Australia, the following applies. U.S. recommendations suggest that Research and Ethical Boards (REBs) should have five or more members, including at least one scientist, one non-scientist and one person not affiliated with the institution. The REB should include people knowledgeable in the law and standards of practice and professional conduct. Special memberships are advocated for handicapped or disabled concerns, if required by the protocol under review. The European Forum for Good Clinical Practice (EFGCP) suggests that REBs include two practicing physicians who share experience in biomedical research and are independent from the institution where the research is conducted; one lay person; one lawyer; and one paramedical professional, e.g. nurse or pharmacist. They recommend that a quorum include both sexes from a wide age range and reflect the cultural make-up of the local community.

The 1996 Australian Health Ethics Committee recommendations were entitled, "Membership Generally of Institutional Ethics Committees". They suggest a chairperson be preferably someone not employed or otherwise connected with the institution. Members should include a person with knowledge and experience in professional care, counselling or treatment of humans; a minister of religion or equivalent, e.g. Aboriginal elder; a layman; a laywoman; a lawyer and, in the case of a hospital-based ethics committee, a nurse. The assignment of philosophers or religious clerics will reflect the importance attached by the society to the basic values involved. An example from Sweden with Torbjorn Tannsjo on a couple of such committees indicates secular trends gaining influence.

Cultural Concerns

Culture differences can create difficult medical ethics problems. Some cultures have spiritual or magical theories about the origins of disease, for example, and reconciling these beliefs with the tenets of Western medicine can be difficult.

Truth-telling

Some cultures do not place a great emphasis on informing the patient of the diagnosis, especially when cancer is the diagnosis. Even American culture did not emphasize truth-telling in a cancer case, up until the 1970s. In American medicine, the principle of informed consent takes precedence over other ethical values, and patients are usually at least asked whether they want to know the diagnosis.

Online Business Practices

The delivery of diagnosis online leads patients to believe that doctors in some parts of the country are at the direct service of drug companies. Finding diagnosis as convenient as what drug still has patent rights on it. Physicians and drug companies are found to be competing for top ten search engine ranks to lower costs of selling these drugs with little to no patient involvement.

Conflicts of Interest

Physicians should not allow a conflict of interest to influence medical judgment. In some cases, conflicts are hard to avoid, and doctors have a responsibility to avoid entering such situations. Unfortunately, research has shown that conflicts of interests are very common among both academic physicians and physicians in practice. The Pew Charitable Trusts has announced the Prescription Project for "academic medical centres, professional medical societies and public and private payers to end conflicts of interest resulting from the $12 billion spent annually on pharmaceutical marketing".

Referral

For example, doctors who receive income from referring patients for medical tests have been shown to refer more patients for medical tests. This practice is proscribed by the American College of Physicians Ethics Manual. Fee splitting and the payments of commissions to attract referrals of patients is considered unethical and unacceptable in most parts of the world - while it is rapidly becoming routine in other countries, like India, where many urban practitioners currently pay a percentage of office-visit charges, lab tests as well as hospital care to unaccredited "quacks", or semi-accredited "practitioners of alternative medicine", who refer the patient. It is tolerated in some areas of US medical care as well.

Vendor Relationships

Studies show that doctors can be influenced by drug company inducements, including gifts and food. Industry-sponsored Continuing Medical Education (CME) programs influence prescribing patterns. Many patients surveyed in one study agreed that physician gifts from drug companies influence prescribing practices. A growing movement among physicians is attempting to diminish the influence of pharmaceutical industry marketing upon medical practice, as evidenced by Stanford University's ban on drug company-sponsored lunches and gifts. Other academic institutions that have banned pharmaceutical industry-sponsored gifts and food include the University of Pennsylvania, and Yale University.

Treatment of Family Members

Many doctors treat their family members. Doctors who do so must be vigilant not to create conflicts of interest or treat inappropriately.

Sexual Relationships

Sexual relationships between doctors and patients can create ethical conflicts, since sexual consent may conflict with the fiduciary responsibility of the physician. Doctors who enter into sexual relationships with patients face the threats of deregistration and prosecution. In the early 1990s it was estimated that 2-9% of doctors had violated this rule Sexual relationships between physicians and patients' relatives may also be prohibited in some jurisdictions, although this prohibition is highly controversial.

Futility

The concept of medical futility has been an important topic in discussions of medical ethics. What should be done if there is no chance that a patient will survive but the family members insist on advanced care? Previously, some articles defined futility as the patient having less than a one percent chance of surviving. Some of these cases wind up in the courts. Advanced directives include living wills and durable powers of attorney for health care. In many cases, the "expressed wishes" of the patient are documented in these directives, and this provides a framework to guide family members and health care professionals in the decision making process when the patient is incapacitated. Undocumented expressed wishes can also help guide decisions in the absence of advanced directives, as in the Quinlan case in Missouri.

"Substituted judgment" is the concept that a family member can give consent for treatment if the patient is unable (or unwilling) to give consent himself. The key question for the decision making surrogate is not, "What would you like to do?", but instead, "What do you think the patient would want in this situation?".

Courts have supported family's arbitrary definitions of futility to include simple biological survival, as in the Baby K case (in which the courts ordered a child born with only a brain stem instead of a complete brain to be kept on a ventilator based on the religious belief that all life must be preserved). In some hospitals, medical futility is referred to as "non-beneficial care." Baby Doe Law establishes state protection for a disabled child's right to life, ensuring that this right is protected even over the wishes of parents or guardians in cases where they want to withhold treatment.

QUALITY OF LIFE (HEALTHCARE)

Quality of life (QOL) is used in healthcare to refer to an individual's emotional, social and physical wellbeing, including their ability to function in the ordinary tasks of living. It is a term used most frequently in the context of medicine and healthcare, where the impact of a disease may reduce "Health-related Quality of Life"

Understanding quality of life is recognized as increasingly important in healthcare, where the relationship between cost and value raises complex problems. For instance, health providers must make economic decisions about access to expensive drugs that may prolong life by a few months, and weight these against alternative uses such as preventative medicine or a surgical bed. Monetary measures alone do not readily apply. In the case of chronic and/or terminal illness where there is no effective treatment or cure, there may be an emphasis on improving HRQoL through interventions such as symptom management, adaptive technology, and palliative care. There is a growing field of research concerned with developing, evaluating and applying quality of life measures within health related research (e.g. within randomized controlled trials), especially Health Services Research. Well-executed HRQoL research informs those tasked with health rationing, is involved in the decision making process of bodies such as the Food and Drug Administration or National Institute for Clinical Excellence, and may be used as an endpoint in clinical trials of experimental therapies.

Initial QoL measures referred to simple assessments of physical abilities by an external rater (e.g.: patient is able to get up, eat and drink, take care of personal hygiene without any help by others), or even to a single measurement (e.g. the angle to which a limb could be flexed).

The current concept of HRQoL acknowledges that subjects put their actual situation in relation to their individual expectation. The latter can vary over time, and react to external influences like long-time disease, family support etc. Patients' and e.g. physicians' rating of the same objective situation have been found to differ significantly. Consequently, HRQoL is nowadays usually assessed using patient questionnaires. These are often multidimensional and cover physical, social, emotional, cognitive, work- or role-related, and possibly spiritual aspects as well as a wide variety of disease related symptoms, therapy induced side-effects, and even the financial impact of medical conditions.

Hundreds of validated QoL questionnaires have been developed: Generic instruments (e.g. SF-36, Short-Form with 36 questions) as well as disease specific instruments (e.g. the LC-13 Lung Cancer module from the EORTC Quality of Life questionnaire library, or the HADS Hospital Anxiety and Depression Scale). Like other psychometric assessment tools, QoL questionnaires should meet certain quality criteria, most importantly with regard to their reliability and validity.

"Improved Quality of Life" is also often advertised for marketing purposes. This is not limited to the medical field; but here, the growing impact of chronic conditions that cannot ultimately be healed, but merely controlled or made bearable, adds to the relevance of the topic.

Frequently Used HRQoL Measures

- Short-Form Health Survey One example of a widely-used questionnaire assessing physical, social, and mental HRQoL, used in clinical trials.
- Manchester Short Assessment of Quality of Life 16-item questionnaire for use in psychiatric populations.
- EQ-5D a simple quality of life questionnaire.

The quality of life ethic refers to an ethical principle which uses assessments of the quality of life that a person can experience or hope to experience as a foundation for making decisions about the continuation or termination of life. It is often used in contrast to or in opposition to the sanctity of life ethic.

TYPES OF LABORATORY

In many countries, there are two main types of labs that process the majority of medical specimens. Hospital laboratories are attached to a hospital, and perform tests on patients. Private (or community) laboratories receive samples from general practitioners, insurance companies, and other health clinics for analysis. These can also be called reference laboratories where more unusual and obscure tests are performed. For extremely specialised tests, samples may go to a research laboratory. A lot of samples are sent between different labs for uncommon tests. It is more cost effective if a particular laboratory specializes in a rare test, receiving specimens (and money) from other labs, while sending away tests it cannot do.

In many countries there are mainly three types of Medical Laboratories as per the types of investigations carried out. Clinical Pathology. Clinical Microbiology & Clinical Biochemistry laboratories. Clinical Pathology: Haematology, Histopathology, Cytology, Routine Pathology. Clinical Microbiology: Bacteriology, Mycobacteriology, Virology, Mycology, Parasitology, Immunology, Serology. Clinical Biochemistry: Biochemical analysis, Hormonal assays etc. Blood Banks:- Blood bank is a separate body. Its laboratory need Microbiological analysis for infectious diseases that may be found in blood. Pathology to observe Blood grouping, Haematology & cross matching reactions. It also involves PRO department for the communication & contact for blood donations etc..

Specimen Processing and Work Flow

Sample processing will usually start with a set of samples and a request form. Typically a set of vacutainer tubes containing blood, or any other specimen, will arrive to the laboratory in a small plastic bag, along with the form. The form and the specimens are given a laboratory number. The specimens will usually all receive the same number, often as a sticker that can be placed on the tubes and form. This label has a barcode that can be scanned by automated analyzers and test requests uploaded from the LIS. Entry of requests onto a laboratory management system involves typing, or scanning (where barcodes are used) in the laboratory number, and entering the patient identification, as well as any tests requested. This allows laboratory machines, computers and staff to know what tests are pending, and also gives a place (such as a hospital department, doctor or other customer) for results to go.

For biochemistry samples, blood is usually centrifuged and serum is separated. If the serum needs to go on more than one machine, it can be divided into separate tubes. Many specimens end up in one or more sophisticated automated analysers, that process a fraction of the sample and return one or more "results". Some laboratories use robotic sample handlers (Laboratory automation) to optimize the workflow and reduce contamination risk and sample handling of the staff. The work flow in a lab is usually heavy from 2:00 am to 10:00 am. Nurses and doctors generally have their patients tested at least once a day with general complete blood counts and chemistry profiles. These orders are then drawn during a morning run by phlebotomists for results to be available in the patient's charts for the attending physicians to consult during their morning rounds. Another busy time for the lab is after 3:00 pm when private practice physician offices are closing. Couriers will pick up specimens that have been drawn throughout the day and deliver them to the lab. Also, couriers will stop at outpatient drawing centres and pick up specimens. These specimens will be processed in the evening and overnight to ensure results will be available the following day.

Laboratory Informatics

Laboratories today are held together by a system of software programs and computers that exchange data about patients, test requests, and test results known as a Laboratory information system or LIS. The LIS is interfaced with the hospital information system. This system enables hospitals and labs to order the correct test requests for each patient, keep track of individual patient or specimen histories, and help guarantee a better quality of results as well as printing hard copies of the results for patient charts and doctors to check.

Result Analysis, Validation and Interpretation

According to ISO 15189 norm, all pathological results must be verified by a competent professional. In some countries staff like clinical scientists do the majority of this work inside the laboratory with abnormal results referred to the relevant pathologist. In others, only medical staff (pathologist or clinical biologist) is concerned by this phase. It can be assisted by some software in order to validate normal or non modified results. Medical staff are sometimes also required in order to explain pathology results to physicians. For a simple result given by phone or for a technical problem it's a medical technologist explaining it to a registered nurse.

Departments in some countries are exclusively directed by a specialized Pathologist, in others a consultant, medical or non-medical, may be the Head of Department. Clinical Scientists have the right to interpret and discuss pathology results in their discipline in many countries, in Europe they are qualified to at least Masters level, may have a PhD and can have an exit qualification equivalent to medical staff e.g. FRC Path in the UK. In France only medical staff (Pharm.D. and M.D. specialized in Anatomical pathology or Clinical biology) can discuss pathological results, clinical scientists are not considered as a part of medical staff.

SCANDAL IN THE CLINICAL LAB INDUSTRY

As medical technology advanced doctors were able to get more and more tests done in shorter and shorter amounts of time. Where in the past a doctor might order a potassium and glucose and it would take hours for the results, now a doctor can order a full chemistry panel of 20 or more different analytes and get the results in under an hour. The results are also much more accurate and reliable now than in the past. Thus, into the 1970s and 1980s the lab became a source of profit within the hospital structure.

Some commercial labs began taking illegal and nefarious actions to increase their income. These practices included medicare and medicaid fraud by performing and billing for tests that the ordering physician never ordered, paying kickbacks to private doctor offices for sending their specimens to these reference labs, and other complicated criminal activity. These kickbacks included donuts, free computers, fax machines, and more. These events culminated mostly in the mid-1990s with the SmithKline Beecham Clinical Laboratory (SBCL) scandal. It is believed SBCL paid at least $325 million in penalties and the industry as a whole paid over $1 billion to insurance and government agencies that were defrauded. Ever since this time, the lab has become a source of expense and loss in the hospital budget (commercial labs have nothing to do with hospitals) and lab medicine's reputation was given a black eye. Now many labs have a compliance officer with mandatory annual meetings about compliance for all employees.

Medical Laboratory Accreditation

Credibility of medical laboratories is paramount to the health and safety of the patients relying on the testing services provided by these labs. The international standard in use today for the accreditation of medical laboratories is ISO 15189 - Medical laboratories - particular requirements for quality and competence.

Accreditation is done by the Joint Commission, AABB, and other state and federal agencies. CLIA 88 or the Clinical Laboratory Improvement Amendments also dictate testing and personnel.

The accrediting body in Australia is NATA, all laboratories must be NATA accredited to receive payment from Medicare. New realities are placing pressures on the healthcare industry, and how patient care is delivered. Rising hospital management costs, an aging population, a shortage of healthcare workers, challenges in accessing services, timely availability of information, issues of safety and quality, and rising consumerism are some of the facts of today's healthcare system. The industry has reached a point of chasm, where they need to decide how services could be delivered more effectively to reduce costs, improve quality, and extend reach. The critical questions facing the industry today include: how can we effectively manage hospitals and provide enhanced services without placing additional burden on a system already pushed to its limits; how can we provide care in a cost-efficient manner at a time when healthcare spending is rising; and how do we most efficiently use our resources and support front-line staff in order to reduce medical errors and enhance quality of care.

These are just a few questions facing the industry. It looks bleak, but there's hope. There are new information technologies available to help. Information technologies that enable immediate, information-rich communications and provide easy-to-use collaborative tools are increasingly becoming a vital part of today's healthcare.

Laboratory medicine is the keystone on which the structure of scientific medicine is erected. A wide variety of laboratory-based disciplines (e.g., histology, hematology, clinical chemistry, Immunology and microbiology) contribute to nearly all of the elements necessary to effectively control infectious and noninfectious diseases. The clinical laboratory is no longer its own limited bionetwork, as it is increasingly integrated with patient care, assisting diagnosis, monitoring therapies and predicting clinical outcomes. A lack of reliable and efficient laboratory service can result in serious consequences for the patients as well as obscuring the true picture of the problem in an entire country.

Clinical laboratories have achieved significant improvements in the provision and quality of diagnostic tests. Automation, commercially produced reagents and computers are providing clinicians with an ever-increasing list of rapid and cost-effective tests. Advances in laboratory medicine have occurred in concert with analytical developments that measure many different molecules with specificity for pathological conditions, and with ever-increasing sensitivity. Such tests have revolutionized clinical diagnosis in ways that were unimaginable even a decade ago. As a consequence, laboratorians and their departments, at least in most developed countries, are expected to meet stringent technical, management and quality-assurance standards.

Laboratory Services in Developing Countries

It is unfortunate that the number and quality of clinical laboratories in developing countries leave a lot to be desired. Although a few top-of-the-line laboratories in these countries compare favorably with those in developed nations, their number is very small. However the vast majority of patients do not have routine access to such laboratories.

In many developing countries, opening a laboratory is as easy as opening a grocery store - or rather, opening a grocery store may be more complicated! A clinical laboratory can be established without requiring permission from any government or professional association. There is no paperwork since there are no regulations governing the management or quality of laboratory practice and in some countries, no license is needed. The factors determining the performance of a clinical laboratory include good equipment, reliable reagents and trained, conscientious staff, but many laboratories compromise on such vital prerequisites. In many cases, retired laboratory technicians and other, often entirely unqualified people, open small clinical laboratories, where standards are not maintained since their knowledge is limited. The managers earn money by using outdated machines, compromising on the reagents and by employing technicians in place of clinical pathologists able to interpret the test results properly and to ensure the achievement of minimal technical standards. Yet the medical laboratory should provide a vital part of the management of any patient – any lapse or mistake in the performance of tests can lead to serious harm whether at the diagnostic stage or in the course of treatment.

Causes of Poor Laboratory Services in Developing Countries

There are numerous causes of poor services, the primary one being failure to follow regulations, or in some cases, to develop relevant regulations. The reasons for this are many and varied but professional laboratory staff as a whole must share the responsibility for tolerating inefficient or obviously incorrect practices. The following factors are especially relevant:

Low Budget: In most developing countries including Egypt, health care is primarily funded from general government revenue without charging the consumers. The expenditure on health is very low to begin with. It is less than one quarter of what developed countries spend and often very much less. Moreover its distribution amongst the various sectors is inequitable. Most funding is spent on high-profile projects in teaching institutions in large urban centres. Laboratory services do not command a high priority.

Scarcity of Laboratory Staff: The tremendous progress in the field of laboratory medicine has made accurate assessment and monitoring the progress of an ailment much easier. The result has been a great rush in demand for laboratory services. It is unfortunate that the availability of laboratory personnel has lagged far behind. In addition, there is significant migration of trained manpower to more profitable markets abroad.

The exact number of clinical laboratory staff working in Egypt, their background and qualifications has not been determined. However, according to one estimate, there are no more than 1500 clinical pathologists, or about 10 per million of the Pakistan population. By contrast, a developed country, such as England, has 109 pathologists per million. Support staff, such as technicians, is in even shorter supply. In Afghanistan there are hardly any at all. In Brazil, until a few years ago, pathologists outnumbered technologists. There is no doubt that a huge gap exists between supply and demand.

Poor Training: The training of pathologists and technicians leaves much to be desired. Most general pathologists have received as little as nine months training in four major subjects. Only in recent years has training been improved to acceptable standards. Similarly, many technicians receive only on-the-job training, with little formal education. The quality of the work of such a body of inadequately trained personnel is bound to be substandard.

Lack of Appropriate Equipment and Infrastructure: Laboratory equipment is mostly manufactured in industrialized countries. It has become increasingly more sophisticated. The procurement officials in developing countries usually buy such fancy gadgetry for purposes of prestige rather than to make full use of its capabilities. There is no infrastructure for maintenance, or even an assured supply of electricity. It is therefore not surprising that developing countries are known as graveyards of equipment. It takes less than one year for some machines to break down in some way and approximately 60-80% of laboratory equipment is estimated to be non-functional.

Lack of Regulatory Mechanisms: There is no license required to establish a clinical laboratory in many developing countries. In Southeast Asian regions of the World Health Organization (WHO), only two out of seven countries had accreditation programs. There are no rules or training requirements for non-pathologist physicians who run or lend their names to laboratories.

Lack of Continuing Education: At present there is almost no provision for continuing education for pathologists. It is usually not required by the institutions that initially award them degrees. The result is that most do not keep up with advances in the field. Yet in such a fast-moving area, it is important that clinical pathologists remain up-to-date with ever-changing technology.

Improvement of *in vitro* Diagnostics in Developing Countries

A number of steps are required of governments as well as professional associations to improve to the current situation:

External Quality Assessment (EQA): A system of EQA including laboratory licensure, accreditation, certification and proficiency testing has to be introduced to provide recognition to those who conform to acceptable standards.

The current international requirements would perhaps be too stringent for the vast majority of existing labs. It may be necessary to evolve a system by which such laboratories are included in a simpler quality assurance program and are gradually brought up to international standards over a period of time.

Training larger numbers of qualified Laboratory Staff: As the number of qualified staff is small, their place is taken up by unqualified non-medicals/untrained physicians. The supply of qualified staff can be increased by providing more training opportunities both within the developing countries themselves and, in some cases, abroad (although this is more expensive and entails the risk of economic migration). It may be helpful to arrange short visits by foreign experts.

Telecommunication: In view of the inadequate supply of trained laboratory staff, telecommunication could provide immediate relief by making expertise available electronically via the Internet or multiple telephone lines in far flung areas. This approach could also be used at an international level for both consultations and training, including continuing education.

Suitable Technologies for Developing Countries: There is a plethora of in vitro diagnostic devices available in more developed countries. Equipment and reagents appropriate to the needs of developing countries should be introduced. A system similar to WHO's essential drug list (essential laboratory tests) has been proposed. Laboratory staff should be trained in such techniques that are less expensive and require less elaborate infra-structure and equipment such that they could be more rapidly and more widely introduced.

The improvement in laboratory services will be a slow process: It is however imperative that a beginning is made so that the suffering of patients is reduced and disease control is brought onto a more rational and firmer footing.

Organize National Structures to Support a Countrywide Laboratory Quality System

National structures capable of supporting a quality system for laboratories at country level will require the following measures: The placement of skilled laboratory scientists/managers with sufficient authority in leadership positions in the ministries of health; Creation of a national laboratory quality office and appointment of a quality officer with authority and responsibility for oversight of national laboratory quality programmes; The allocation of adequate financial resources to ensure compliance with national quality programmes.

ESTABLISH NATIONAL LABORATORY QUALITY STANDARDS

International efforts are under way to develop health laboratory standards that help to ensure quality.

These efforts should be supported as follows: Each country should establish its own set of standards according to country-specific needs based on internationally agreed standards. National laboratory standards need to take into account local factors, including any pertinent regulations, organization of the country's laboratory system(s), and resource constraints.

It is recommended that countries with limited resources consider taking a staged approach, where principal requirements for all are stated in the national laboratory standards as a minimum requirement while more advanced and national reference laboratories are encouraged to aim at meeting internationally accepted standards such as ISO 15189.

Implement Major Laboratory Quality System Programmes

Many activities associated with quality assurance must be carried out by local laboratories, but assistance and oversight will be required at the national level. The following activities should be planned at a national level, with help and input from laboratories throughout the country, to:

- establish and revise national quality standards;
- ensure that laboratory facilities and infrastructure are adequate and properly maintained for all testing being performed;
- ensure safety in all health laboratory facilities to protect workers within the laboratory, visitors to the facility and the general public at large;
- establish long-range plans for ensuring adequate and sustainable numbers of properly trained personnel for conducting laboratory operations;
- apply appropriate quality systems to all parts of laboratory management and operations, including the procurement
- process for supplies and equipment;
- develop national resources for ensuring internal quality control and for external quality assessment;
- develop a process for monitoring laboratory performance improvement;
- encourage the development of a structured advisory network for laboratories.

5

Health Care Administration

Health care administrators take care of the business side of medicine. Health care administration is the business side of the medical field. People in this field manage hospitals, nursing homes and rehabilitation care facilities. Specialists may focus on managing specific business functions within the medical office. Functions such as billing, medical records or human resources management are examples of specialization within health care administration.

Education

According to the U.S. Department of Labor, Occupational Outlook Handbook for 2010-2011, you will need a master's degree in either public health, public administration, long-term care administration, health sciences or health services administration to begin a career in health care administration. Some medical practices will also accept a bachelor's degree for entry-level positions. To obtain a master's degree, you must first complete a bachelor's degree from an accredited college. Requirements vary among graduate schools, and you should plan your undergraduate work to meet admission requirements for the graduate school of your choice.

License

License requirements vary depending on your chosen specialty. For example, the American Association of Health Care Administration Management (AAHAM) offers classes and testing for Certified Patient Account Manager (CPAM), and Certified Clinic Account Manager (CCAM). The CPAM certification is for people specializing in billing, credit and collections, accounts receivable management, and admissions and registration.

The CCAM certificate focus on patient communication and registration, credit and collections, billing and accounts receivable management. These exams are compared to the CPA test for accountants, and the bar exam for lawyers. Other professional exams offered by AAHAM prove technical proficiency. These are the Certified Patient Account Technician (CPAT), and Certified Clinic Account Technician (CCAT).

ECONOMIC IMPLICATIONS FOR THE HOSPITAL OF THE FUTURE

The High Cost of Doing Business

In 2007, the national expenditure on health care was over $2.2 trillion, or $7,500 per U.S. resident. Health care spending accounts for 16.2 per cent of Gross Domestic Product (GDP). More than onethird of national health spending is for hospital care, compared to approximately 20 per cent for physician services and 10 per cent for pharmaceuticals.

While health care costs are rising globally, in no country are costs rising at the high rate of those of the U.S. Overall, U.S. per capita health care spending is more than 50 per cent higher than any other country. Among the most significant reasons for this contrast are higher income and higher medical prices in the U.S. Indeed, the U.S. pays much higher prices for pharmaceuticals, hospital stays and physician visits. For its level of investment, the U.S. does not receive a more favourable rate of return as far as higher quality care, patient satisfaction or population health status compared to other industrialized nations.

Higher health care costs that are borne by health care purchasers, payers, and consumers are becoming untenable. As a result, health care purchasers are focusing on health benefit cost containment strategies, mainly by shifting more of the cost burden to employees. Job-based health insurance premiums rose 10-times faster than incomes from 2001 to 2005, according to a report from the Robert Wood Johnson Foundation. The amount employees paid for family coverage rose 30 per cent, while their incomes rose by three per cent. Fewer private- sector businesses offer coverage (-30,000) and as a result, 4.1 million fewer employees are working in private-sector jobs that offer health insurance. Overall, 2.4 million fewer people have private health insurance, a drop of six per cent. Year to year more people are uninsured.

Today, that figure stands at approximately 47 million people. Meanwhile, public health insurance programmes are experiencing the squeeze of the current economic scenario. High health care costs, a poorly performing U.S. economy, diminished tax revenue, a booming Medicare-eligible generation, as well as growing ranks of uninsured are factors in the expected insolvency of the Medicare programme by 2019.

More Red Than Rosy

While many hospitals are today enjoying relative prosperity – in one survey, hospital systems reported an increase in patient revenues of nearly 8.5 per cent in 2007 from the previous year — the conditions upon which these gains are made are expected to dramatically change in the coming years. And, while some hospitals experience healthy profit margins, an uncomfortable number of hospitals continue to be unprofitable.

There is a growing gap between have and have-not hospitals that may very well widen as the future unfolds. Hospitals are not invulnerable to current economic conditions. While health care has long been thought to be "recession-proof" because of an endless supply of sick patients and reliance on government payment, health care organizations are as vulnerable to the tightened credit market as any industry.

According to a report in *Modern Health care,* even before the economy started to falter this year, hospital and health system bond rating downgrades were on the upswing, while upgrades were on the downswing. In fact, about 50 per cent of shortterm, acute-care hospitals are either insolvent or near insolvency, according to a recent report from Alvarez and Marshal Health care Industry Group. Financial issues are mainly arising from the instability of funding sources, including government subsidies and charitable contributions. Moreover, hospital capital expenses are underfunded by up to $20 billion. By and large, many hospitals are able to achieve a positive bottom-line through cost-shifting – subsidizing services that do not cover costs with more favourable remunerative services. For treating Medicare patients, hospitals receive $.91 of every dollar expended; for Medicaid patients they receive $.86 per dollar.

Uncompensated care accounts for approximately six per cent of hospital costs on average – in 2006 that amounted to $30 billion. Yet, from private payers, hospitals receive $1.22 for every dollar spent. Hospitals depend on having robust numbers of privately insured patients in order to be able to treat the under- and uninsured and still remain in the black. This scenario will be increasingly difficult to sustain.

With the demographic trend pointing to a growing elderly population, hospitals can expect to have more Medicare patients. Absent any major health reform, with the continuing decline in employer-sponsored insurance and unabated growth in the numbers of uninsured, hospitals can expect more Medicaid patients and uncompensated care. In essence, there will be more competition for the fewer patients to whom costs may be shifted. There is another wrinkle in the cross-subsidy fabric.

In order to address escalating health care costs, stakeholders are demanding transparency of the costs and quality of care. For its part, the federal government has been taking steps to encourage price and quality transparency as one way to spur competition and encourage value-based health care purchasing decisions. An August 2006 Executive Order requires federal agencies that administer or sponsor health programmes to make information available to consumers on the quality and costs of services provided by doctors and hospitals.

The Executive Order also requires agencies and their contractors to promote the use of interoperable health care information technology products so that data can easily be shared. The Order further requires federal agencies to offer health insurance programmes that reward consumers who choose health care providers based on value and quality. Based on the Executive Order, the Health and Human Services Secretary launched the Value- Driven Health Care Initiative, the agenda for which includes four "cornerstones" – transparency of quality information, transparency of pricing information, promotion of health information technology adoption, and creation of incentive mechanisms to promote quality and efficiency.

Transparency of pricing will likely foster what is now absent in health care – a price-sensitive consumer. While it is unclear how hospital pricing – and all of its irrational complexity – will be translated for consumer understanding, the net effect may be a flattening of health care pricing, and diminished opportunity for cross-subsidization to cover money-losing procedures and patients.

Transparency in both price and quality may, however, boost the market position of specialty hospitals. Specialty hospitals act as "focused factories," serving a subset of patients to perform specific procedures, such as cardiac care and orthopedic surgery. As such, they focus on delivering well-paying services to an insured pool of patients.

Without departments such as emergency, trauma and intensive care, specialty hospitals are free of the regulatory and social obligations that general hospitals are held to. And, with high margins, focused expertise and high volume, specialty hospitals can be very competitive on price and quality.

The market and financial advantages of specialty hospitals have not gone unnoticed, and even spurred a moratorium on any new development for awhile. Now that the moratorium has been lifted, the Centres for Medicare and Medicaid (CMS) has proposed correcting inequalities by lowering the reimbursement rate for the diagnostic-related group (DRG) codes that attracted specialty hospital business in the first place.

This could be an important leveller since surgery and procedure-related treatment has long been known to attract a higher financial reward than providing medical care, and has therefore created its own set of incentives. This action, though, will not require specialty hospitals to share in providing care that is solely for the public good.

Further, it will lower the reimbursement rate that all hospitals receive for performing these same services and further erode future hospital revenue that provides coverage for mission-related services. In the meantime, hospitals are readying for "no pay for preventable events."

As of October 2008, Medicare no longer reimburses hospitals for a growing list of hospital-acquired conditions, such as surgical-site infection and pressure ulcers, as part of its Value-Based Purchasing Initiative. Private-sector payers are quickly following suit.

CMS is also looking at ways to equalize payment by using hospital costs rather than charges to set rates. It recently began adjusting payment to better recognize severity of illness and the cost of treating Medicare patients by increasing payments for some services and decreasing payments for others. Fiscal pressures will also keep the pressure on future Medicare and Medicaid provider reimbursements, and it is expected that CMS will continue to seek more avenues to not pay for "preventable conditions" that occur in health care organizations.

Beyond Borders

High health care costs and inadequate access to specialized care are fuelling fast growth in medical tourism. Would-be patients in developed countries are travelling thousands of miles – most often to India and Thailand — to receive high-quality care at dramatically lower costs and with no wait. Medical tourism is now a multi-billion-dollar industry.

In years past, a medical tourist was someone seeking services that were not covered by health plans, such as cosmetic surgery. Today, a medical tourist is as likely to be seeking full or partial joint replacement, cardiac surgery or even stem cell therapy. Typically, U.S. citizens that have gone abroad have either been uninsured or underinsured and therefore, price-sensitive to the cost of their needed surgeries.

The profile of the U.S. medical tourist is changing, however, as selfinsured employers and third-party payers are beginning to add coverage for treatment received abroad as a means to lower their own costs. Rather than wait months or years for an elective surgery, patients in some European countries are crossing borders for more immediate care. As a result, some European Union (EU) countries, such as the United Kingdom (UK), are reimbursing patients for the cost of acute care received outside of their country of origin on a case-by-case basis.

For some European countries, shortening waiting lists may mean exporting patients to elsewhere in the EU, or it may mean importing health care services to bolster the volume of services provided and quicken turnaround times. The phenomenon of the medical tourist seeking complex and necessary care for their well-being outside of their own "health jurisdiction" raises important concerns for the hospital of the future. On one hand, such medical tourism may represent an elaboration of an individual's right to choose. But, it may also exemplify the failure of a society to fulfil its social contract with its citizens.

A global health care marketplace is an increasing competitive threat for U.S. hospitals. A new study from Deloitte finds that the number of patients leaving the U.S. for medical treatment is growing at a faster rate than the number coming for treatment. The study projects that U.S. health care providers will lose nearly $16 billion in revenue this year to outbound medical travel. That figure is expected to grow to $68 billion by 2010, a 325 per cent rise. Hospitals are "flattening" for a variety of reasons in addition to globe-trekking patients.

The outsourcing of services to offshore entities, such as for radiology, is another way in which hospitals are becoming more global and horizontally configured. But, there are domestic factors that are influencing the flattening of hospitals, as well. Specialty hospitals "disaggregate" hospital services that were once integral to the hospital. In response, hospitals are striking up partnerships with physicians in these ventures so that they can retain some share of the market.

The Home Team

Despite the impact of globalization and "disaggregation," hospitals have a mission to fulfil to society. No new specialty hospitals or offshore services are being developed to serve the poor, elderly and under- or uninsured. With the coming squeeze on health care pricing and increased competition, hospitals will need to adapt. They will have to learn to do more with less by squeezing out inefficiencies in care delivery. Without the prospect of higher reimbursement rates, hospitals will have to reduce their costs in order to achieve equilibrium in the ratio of payments received to costs expended.

There are some seemingly irrational health care expenditures, that on the surface, cry out for a more efficient approach. End-of-life care is an example. In the U.S., highest per capita health care expenditure occurs in the last months of life.

Several other countries perform markedly better by this measure and spend less on care at the end of life. However, "to do as they do" is not as easy as it seems. Differences in social norms, laws, regulations and litigation trends are among the reasons why there are no easy answers to this complex problem.

The national focus on health care cost containment strategies and increasingly unstable sources of funding are providing strong influence on hospitals to drive out waste and inefficiencies.

Hospitals are increasingly relying on quality improvement tools such as Lean and Six Sigma to create efficient, high-quality care processes. In addition to improved patient safety and higher quality, many organizations are experiencing cost savings through these efforts.

For whom these costs are saved remains an issue. Many of the savings, such as those derived from processes that reduce utilization of higher cost services, accrue to health care payers and are revenue losers for hospitals.

A realigned and rational payment structure that provides incentives for waste reduction must accompany efforts aimed at creating an efficient – and equally effective – hospital industry.

New payment schemes, such as pay-for-performance, are providing hospitals with incentive to focus on specific priorities and maximize quality related to the various measures these programmes track. These programmes will increasingly focus on creating efficiencies in care delivery. But, more alignment of economic incentives with quality goals – such as improved care for the chronically ill — is needed. The key challenge for the hospital of the future is to be able to fulfil its social mission in an environment of constrained federal payment while also investing in new technologies and capital improvements.

TECHNOLOGY FOR THE PROVISION OF CARE

More Than the Building

- "...no matter what your profession – doctor, lawyer, architect, accountant — ...you better be good at the touchy-feely service stuff, because anything that can be digitized can be outsourced to either the smartest or the cheapest producer, or both... 'Everyone has to focus on what exactly is their value-add.'" — from The World is Flat by Thomas Friedman

With digital technology, radiologists in Bangalore, India do not have to come to the U.S. to practice, U.S. radiology films can go to them. Even more profoundly, digital technology is changing the locus of care delivery and allowing for more care — care that may fall under the umbrella of the hospital — to occur outside of the hospital's walls. In the U.S., the Department of Veterans' Affairs (VA) is on the cutting edge of using digital technology to better meet the needs of a growing number of military veterans, both those who are reaching their senior years and those newly returned from current conflicts.

The VA's national Care Coordination Home Telehealth (CCHT) Programme was first implemented in 2004 to bring about a transition of institutionally based care and chronic care management from hospitals and clinics to patients' own homes when indicated and appropriate. Telehealth applications combined with disease management methods and a comprehensive electronic health record (EHR) support VA care coordinators to remotely monitor patients and thereby enhance and extend care and management.

The emphasis of CCHT is on patient self-management and providing a programme of care, rather than the traditional episodic approach to care. Remote monitoring technologies enable disease management questions and objective data – for instance, blood glucose levels of a diabetic patient – to be uploaded to their Electronic Health Record (EHR) daily.

Care coordinators, who are usually nurses and social workers, use these data to prioritize who among their patients needs active care management. CCHT enables a single care coordinator to support a caseload of between 120 and 150 patients depending on case mix. In selected patients, videoconferencing capabilities even allow for virtual physician office visits in the home, which is especially beneficial for patients living in remote areas.

This application of technology is not intended to replace the high-touch aspect of care delivery. Because of the heavy emphasis on disease management and vital sign monitoring, CCHT helps to reduce disease complications, and allows patients and caregivers to recognize sooner when a doctor's visit or a hospital admission may be necessary. Currently, the CCHT programme supports the care of 33,883 patients in their own homes.

Outcomes data from a cohort of 17,025 patients showed a 20 per cent reduction in hospital admissions and a 25 per cent reduction in hospital bed days of care. The efficiencies and quality improvements gained through the VA's CCHT programme are helping the VA to serve more patients and change the location of care in accordance with patient preferences. Veteran patients receiving CCHT care have a mean satisfaction score of 86 per cent. CCHT is part of a larger transition in the location of care for patients that is making care more accessible and convenient for veteran patients.

In 1995, the VA system had 50,000 hospital beds; today it has 18,000 with the addition of over 1,000 sites of care in local communities that provide primary and ambulatory care. In the intervening period, the VA has become markedly more efficient with a relatively modest increase in clinical staffing, but a dramatic rise in the number of patients served – increasing from 2.5 million to 5 million in the same time frame. Like its counterparts in the non-federal health system, the VA has to do more with less. The migration of care from the hospital bed and physician office to the home that is allowed through technology invites the redefinition of the hospital.

Rather than being defined by its number of beds, the "value-add" of the hospital of the future may be its intellectual property. A hospital will be able to lend its expertise to the care of a patient located in a vastly different place than where its facility is located. As an integrated, single-payer system, standardization and innovation is perhaps easier to achieve in the VA system than in hospitals and other health care providers that operate in a more fragmented environment.

Implementation of new models of care like the CCHT involve changes in clinical practice, technology infrastructure and business processes. Given the underlying need to care for greater numbers of patients with chronic disease, telehealth and remote patient monitoring could have the same evolutionary impact outside of the VA as it has had within.

Mighty I.T.

At the core of the VA's Care Coordination Programme is a comprehensive electronic health record system that is in standard use across VA health delivery sites, including remotely delivered care in the home. In fact, the VA has the largest enterprisewide health information system in the U.S. Outside of the VA, only approximately 11 per cent of non-federal hospitals and 12 per cent of physician practices have implemented comprehensive electronic health records.

Many other countries, including the United Kingdom, Germany, Denmark, Australia and Canada have moved ahead of the U.S. in deploying health information technology. In fact, the U.S. lags a dozen years behind other industrialized countries in health information technology (HIT) adoption. In all of the countries that have implemented national HIT programmes, the costs have been paid by the government and health insurers, and not by the health care providers.

These countries have viewed their investment in HIT as a public good, the benefits of which – reduced costs and improved quality — will mainly accrue to health care payers and patients. Implementation challenges in these countries are also far easier to overcome given their relatively simple payer structures and centralized decision-making capacity as compared to the U.S. With fewer payers – and in some cases, such as in the U.K., centralized vendor selection — the ability to standardize nomenclature and build an interoperable platform is made easier. In the U.S., attempts by payers, coalitions and oversight bodies to influence the rate of adoption of HIT have had mixed results. Following the IOM's release of *To Err is Human* in 1999, the Leapfrog Group – a consortium of large employers – established its first "leaps" in patient safety for hospitals serving their employees to meet.

Among this first set of standards was the requirement that hospitals implement computerized physician order entry (CPOE) systems. Although this requirement came in 2000, still only about five per cent of all U.S. hospitals have a CPOE system. Clearly, this leap has fallen short. Leapfrog attributes this to the sheer cost of implementing CPOE and resistance by physicians. For its part in advancing the adoption of electronic health records, the federal government created the Office of the National Coordinator for Health Information Technology (ONC) within the Department of Health and Human Services (HHS).

ONC's primary purpose is to coordinate the development of standards that will allow for interoperability between systems, and a national health information network through which health information can be exchanged. In 2005, HHS created the American Health Information Community (AHIC).

This federal advisory committee includes representatives from both the private and public sectors and is charged to provide recommendations to HHS on making health records digital and interoperable, as well as capable of protecting the privacy of patient information. HHS is now in the process of transitioning the AHIC to a successor organization under funding to the Brookings Institution and LMI Consulting.

It is envisioned that the AHIC-2 will not start from whole cloth, but will learn from and enhance the work of the existing AHIC's efforts to promote electronic interchange of information. AHIC-2 is expected to be even more inclusive than AHIC and may also involve some regional loci for its work.

In the meantime, HHS has launched demonstration projects through which it provides financial incentives for health care practitioners to use HIT. The Medicare Care Management Demonstration, in part, provides additional payment to physicians who use an EHR certified by the Certification Commission for Health care Information Technology (CCHIT) to electronically submit performance data on 26 measures.

The most recent demonstration project allows CMS to make bonus payments to small physician practices that use a certified EHR for clinical documentation and e-prescribing. Payments are determined based on the practices' performance on specific quality measures.

It may be that many hospitals still need to be convinced of the value of HIT. While there is a strong evidence base supporting claims that such HIT systems yield significant benefit for the safety and quality of health care, there has been insufficient research conducted to support the return on investment from HIT. And, the level of required investment can be substantial.

Initial implementation costs may range from several hundred thousand dollars for initial implementation in a physician office to millions in a community hospital to tens of millions of dollars in an academic medical center.

Annual maintenance of the systems can cost tens of thousands to several million dollars. Many are also wary of the work flow disruptions that a full-scale IT implementation can cause. Enhancing work flow and care process redesign needs to be part and parcel of the implementation plan. Failure to do so can serve to codify already broken or defective care processes. Involving clinical staff who will be using the technology – at the patient's bedside, in the office, pharmacy, lab and home – in its development and providing followon training are key to its success. Issues of interoperability remain generally unsolved as of today.

While health care policymakers and standards bodies hammer out solutions for achieving interoperability of systems that will allow for data sharing between separate entities, many health care providers see this as a reason to wait to invest in HIT. Unsolved issues around data privacy and fear of system obsolescence further fuel their hesitancy. In the meantime, lack of interoperability between HIT systems and medical devices that have an HIT component – such as hospital beds that take readings of vital signs but do not integrate with the EHR – slow the workflow of care providers.

Indeed, nurses are often the "integrators" of patient information between HIT systems. As new technologies are added to the workplace, it is essential that they be labour-saving in order to conserve already stretched professional resources.

Buy or Beware

With a well-funded biotechnology industry, new technologies are constantly being created with the hope of creating a new disease market or need. This constant barrage of technology purchasing decisions may be difficult to navigate since any new purchase creates an opportunity to increase costs – and waste — in the system. Adding certain new technologies into the health care work place can be very disruptive to work flow and exacerbate inefficiencies. Technologies that are not integrative with other technologies add very little value to the patient's care and the health care worker's practice.

With a plethora of cutting-edge information and clinical technology purchasing decisions to be made under a tight budget, health care professionals could use an objective authority to help guide their value-based investments. From 1974-1995, the Congressional Office of Technology Assessment (OTA) provided Congress with objective analysis of contemporary issues involving science and technology.

OTA reports were highly authoritative and well respected. Similar functions in other countries were even modeled after the OTA. But, these reports were sometimes unpopular, especially when their conclusions ran counter to the interests of affected industries.

The OTA lost its funding in 1995. The loss of the OTA has left a void. In 2004, a new bill to re-establish some of the capabilities of the OTA was defeated; however, many feel that Congress would benefit from expert analyses of many of the complex scientific and technological issues that are often a source of debate. Though there are private-sector sources for information to support technology decision-making, the OTA served as a public source for much-needed information.

ACHIEVEMENT OF PATIENT-CENTRED CARE

The Main Point

- At Cincinnati Children's Hospital, family members are included in patient rounds in the pediatric intensive care unit and the hospital encourages family-centred rounds on all of its clinical units. MCG Health System in Augusta, Georgia relies on its Patient and Family Advisory Council to inform the physical design of its care environments and even its compliance with Joint Commission National Patient Safety Goals. Across its various advisory councils, the University of Washington Medical Center recruits patient and family member volunteers to interview and select residency candidates, and to develop patient educations materials and other supportive programmes for patients and family members. As a result of revelations concerning patient safety, hospitals have had to look inward at practices, policies and even the cultures and attitudes that are prevalent in their delivery settings. In so doing, there is now renewed emphasis and acceptance that it is the patient who is at the center of care. Not only is the patient the main point, but the patient has the greatest stake in their care and as such, should be respected as an equal partner in their care. The elevation of the patient to partner is not a ceremonial title bestowed for a "feel good" moment, but has significant implications for the quality and safety of patient care. When it comes to their health, patients often do not act alone on their own behalf, but their health care decisions are intertwined with those closest to them – their family members or others to whom they are emotionally tied. Family, then, is the third part of the triumvirate in the health care partnership. The Institute for Family-Centred Care defines the core concepts of patient-centred care as: *Dignity and Respect* – Health care practitioners listen to and honour patient and family perspectives and choices. Patient and family knowledge, values, beliefs and cultural backgrounds are incorporated into the planning and delivery of care.

- *Information Sharing* – Health care practitioners communicate and share complete and unbiased information with patients and families in ways that are affirming and useful. Patients and families receive timely, complete, and accurate information in order to effectively participate in care and decision-making.
- *Participation* – Patients and families are encouraged and supported in participating in care and decision-making at the level they choose.
- *Collaboration* – Patients and families are also included on an institution-wide basis. Health care leaders collaborate with patients and families in policy and programme development, implementation, and evaluation; in health care facility design; and in professional education, as well as in the delivery of care.

Another resource for patient-centred care guidance is Planetree. Planetree is a non-profit organization that provides education and information to health care organizations to facilitate the delivery of patient-centred care. Planetree's Patient-Centred Care Designation Programme recognizes hospitals that meet its criteria for patient-centred care.

These criteria have been compiled based upon the experiences of hospitals who have achieved patient-centred care, as well as the feedback of patients.

The criteria are used to measure organizations' structures and functions that support patient-centred care concepts; human interactions; patient education and community access to information; family involvement; nutrition; the architecture and interior design of the healing environment, art programmes; spirituality and diversity; integrative therapies, community health; and measurement.

Nothing Without Me

Engaging patients in their care has real implications for the quality and safety of patient care. A large study of adult patients with chronic or serious conditions who were engaged in a collaborative care model had better control of their blood pressure, blood glucose levels, and serum cholesterol than patients who had less confidence either in their doctors or their ability to care for themselves.

Another study of patients hospitalized for acute myocardial infarction found that patients who rated hospitals poorly on Picker Institute measures of patient-centred care had poorer health outcomes than those who experienced more patient-centred care.

The experiences of MCG Health System in Augusta, Georgia attests to the prospects for patient-centred care in improving quality and safety. In 2003, the health system redesigned its intensive care unit for neuroscience patients to allow patients' families to stay with them at all times.

The observances of family members were valued by the unit's clinical staff. Owing to these insights and improved communications, medication errors in the unit decreased 62 per cent, length of stay decreased 50 per cent, and the staff vacancy rate fell from 7.5 per cent to zero. Patient satisfaction ratings increased from the tenth percentile to the 95th. In the words of an MCG staff member, the families "helped us help their loved ones."

Engagement of patients and families empowers patients to participate in care decisions, provide self-care, and protect themselves from potential harm. In fact, The Joint Commission's National Patient Safety Goal 13 specifically requires health care organization staff to encourage patients' active involvement in their care as a patient safety strategy. Goal 13 further requires staff to identify ways in which the patient and his or her family can report concerns about safety and encourage them to do so.

The rationale for this goal states that "communication with the patient and family about all aspects of care, treatment, and services is an important characteristic of a culture of safety. When the patient knows what to expect, he or she is more aware of possible errors and choices.

The patient can also be an important source of information about potential adverse events and hazardous conditions." The aspect of patient empowerment within patient-centred care has led to the notion of "nothing about me, without me."

Momentum

In addition to Joint Commission standards and safety goals, other organizational and professional accrediting bodies increasingly emphasize the importance of engaging patients in the delivery of care. In the U.S., the inclusion of information pertaining to patients' perspectives of care on the CMS Web site, *Hospital Compare*, provides a powerful incentive for hospitals to better meet the expectations of patients.

The survey – called H-CAHPS – addresses issues such as the quality of nurse and physician communications with patients, discharge instructions, and medication education. In the international arena, the U.K. National Health Service (NHS) is requiring its hospitals and primary care clinics to engage patients and family in quality improvement efforts. Across Canada, patients are being similarly engaged.

The World Health Organization (WHO) has also made patient and family engagement in patient safety improvement a major priority of its World Alliance for Patient Safety, launched in 2004. Patients and families are also driving momentum. Several patient advocacy organizations, such as Partnerships for Patient Safety (p4ps) and PULSE are organized around the goal of advancing patient centred care and improving patient safety. Social momentum for patient-centred care is also likely to increase with the growth of consumerdirected health plans and health savings accounts (HSAs). Such health plans increase the health care consumers' responsibility for making value-based health care purchasing decisions.

Technology is another momentum-building factor. The advent of personal health records (PHRs) will provide patients with "point and click" access to their own health records as well as enhanced communications capabilities with their care providers. Technology that is allowing patients to receive higher levels of care in their homes underscores the need for a patient-centred approach to care, especially as their role as "partner" in care delivery becomes a 24/7 endeavour.

These patients and families need personalized education and training, as well as a professional support system so that the transition to home-based care is safe and effective for all involved.

Custom and Culture

While momentum is certainly building and the concept of patient-centred care is widely embraced, much is still getting lost in the execution. There are barriers, not the least of which is the heightened need for patient education when practitioners seemingly have less time to spend with patients – ala the 10-minute office visit.

There are also issues of health literacy – in the U.S. alone, nearly half the population lacks the skills necessary to obtain, process, and understand basic health information and services needed to make appropriate health decisions. The focus in patient-centred care on transparency can make hospital risk managers uneasy. Yet, several studies have revealed that what patients really want – open disclosure, communications and collaboration – nurtures, rather than harms, patient and caregiver relationships.

It is also important to underscore what patient-centred care is not. In some countries, the term is a euphemism for a lower tier of care, where the de facto caregiver is the family – not in partnership with practitioners – but on their own. There are other cultural differences to patient-centred care. In Thai culture, the family will stay at the patient's bedside round-the-clock and help with feeding and personal support. But, neither a Thai patient nor family member will generally participate in decision- making — that is the province of the physician, whose level of education is held in high esteem.

In any country, it is also important to recognize that not every patient wants to be a partner in their care, nor do they wish their family to be. The level of partnership may vary – some patients may wish to be 50/50 partners, others may wish for much less. For the hospital of the future, care must be increasingly customized to the personal expectations, cultural beliefs and traditions, and language needs of the patient. In eliciting patients' needs and expectations of their care, hospitals may need to perform an intake interview that covers these topics at the time of admission.

Instilling patient-centred care is not just about changing policies and practices; it is about changing culture, which is never easily done. For staff to be empathetic to patients, the hospital must also have an empathetic culture for staff. Staff members need to be supported through systems that protect them from harm – and from doing harm. In the absence of such cultures and work environments, staff members may become overburdened and increasingly demoralized.

To achieve a culture that is patient-centred and supportive of staff, hospital leadership and staff must share common beliefs and values. Coming to these common beliefs and values may be the hardest part of achieving cultural change.

Serving the Underserved

In the U.S., there are specific populations who are the least likely to receive patient-centred care. For minority groups and the poor, disparities in health care quality and access persist. The 2007 National

Health care Disparities Report issued by the Agency for Health care Research and Quality reveals that, overall, disparities have not been reduced despite the growing body of evidence of their existence, though there have been small gains. Positive examples include the adequacy of hemodialysis for Black and for White patients, and the hospital admission rate among Hispanics and the poor and their White.

These small gains are offset by the persistence of wide disparities in health care quality that have resulted in disproportionate numbers of minorities and poor who have AIDS, lower immunization rates, and lack access to prenatal care, among other examples of unequal treatment. Sometimes it is the provenance of their illness that creates disparate access to quality health care for patients.

Mentally ill patients are perhaps the most underserved patient population today. A report from a special commission to President Bush claims that half of Americans who need mental health care are not getting it, even if they have sought it. Mainly due to a payment system that does not support the provision of psychiatric care, many hospital- based and free-standing psychiatric services have closed or reduced their number of beds.

In fact, from 1995 to 1999, the number of psychiatric beds in this country shrunk by 38 per cent. All the while, demand for inpatient psychiatric care has climbed, leaving the mentally ill often with nowhere else to turn but to the hospital emergency department for care.

In fact, emergency departments across the country report an influx of mentally ill patients coming through their doors. With so few alternatives to place these patients in a psychiatric bed, the emergency department often holds these patients for hours, even days. Though the roots of the problem began more than a decade ago, it is a problem that worsens year to year. In a 2007 AHA survey, 42 per cent of hospitals reported an increase in boarding behavioural health patients in the emergency department. The boarding of psychiatric patients brings its own particular strain and costs. Crowded emergency departments, with staff and resources stretched thin, cannot provide the intense care and monitoring psychiatric patients in crisis need, which is best provided in an appropriate setting and by specially trained health care workers.

On The Rise

Today, half of all hospitalized patients have one or more chronic condition, such as diabetes, heart disease and asthma. The prevalence of chronic illness is expected to steadily increase. By 2030, it is estimated that 171 million people will have at least one chronic illness. By this same year, older adults will account for more than 20 per cent of the population.

While older adults are expected to live longer, this will not be without personal health challenges. More than 75 per cent of adults over age 65 suffer from at least one chronic condition, and many have multiple conditions. Among current Medicare beneficiaries, 20 per cent have five or more chronic conditions. Aging is not the only factor driving the burgeoning ranks of the chronically ill.

Owing to its significantly higher rates of obesity and smoking, the U.S. has a significantly higher rate of associated diseases – such as diabetes, hypertension and heart disease – than European countries. According to the Centres for Disease Control and Prevention (CDC), 80 per cent of diabetes, heart disease and stroke could be eliminated through reductions in smoking and obesity. There is widespread recognition that care for the chronically ill in the U.S. is falling short. An oftcited report from RAND indicates that the chronically ill receive approximately half of recommended care.

At the root of this issue is the predominant organization of the health delivery and payment system to support the diagnosis and treatment of acute, or episodic, conditions. Patients with chronic illness, especially those with multiple conditions, often receive care from multiple providers and take many medications.

Because this care is uncoordinated, patients may experience duplicative services and testing, avoidable hospitalization, and adverse drug events. As a result, care is often fragmented, ineffective and costly for people with chronic diseases. Optimal care for people with chronic diseases involves coordinated, continuous treatment by a multidisciplinary team of health care professionals.

These patients need education and tools to support self-management, and connections to community resources for their social, mental health and home health needs.

For the hospital of the future, providing patientcentered care means better meeting the needs of all of its patients, including the underserved, the aged and the chronically ill who will fill its beds in greater numbers.

Patient-Centred Transformation

To increase their reliability in delivering patientcentered care, hospitals can turn to the process improvement tools — such as Six Sigma and Lean, among others — that have proved effective for transforming other industries. A glimpse of that transformation can be seen at hospitals like Virginia Mason Medical Center in Seattle, which has applied these tools to improve the quality of care for patients with low back pain and other conditions, increase adherence to evidence-based care, and decrease costs.

In ThedaCare hospitals in southern Wisconsin, application of these methods to general medical units has allowed the hospitals to reduce medication errors, the average amount of time these patients are hospitalized, and the fees charged for certain procedures. New York-Presbyterian Hospital used these tools to reduce average length of stay for patients undergoing cardiac and orthopedic procedures, reduce medication errors and patient falls, and increase patient satisfaction rates.

THE STAFFING CHALLENGE

Wide and Deep

Hospitals rank second as a source of private-sector jobs nationwide. In urban areas, hospitals are among the top ten employers, and are often the largest employer in rural areas. Health care, broadly, contributed more jobs to the economy than any other industry in the last several years.

Still, the demand for certain health professionals outstrips supply. Workforce shortages have persistently plagued hospitals over the last several years. In 2007, as well as in previous years, it has ranked in the top five issues confronting hospital CEOs according to a poll conducted by the American College of Health care Executives. Staffing problems are widespread across health care professions.

Therapists – physical, occupational and speech – are in especially short supply and increasingly difficult to recruit from year to year. Vacancy rates for these positions exceeded 11 per cent by year-end 2006. Registered nurses, pharmacists, nursing assistants, licensed practical nurses, and laboratory and imaging technicians all have vacancy rates in the range of six per cent for technicians to eight per cent for RNs.

There is also growing national concern over shortages of physicians – already a problem in several states – that is expected to worsen as demand outstrips supply. By 2020, the U.S. may be short 85,000 physicians.

It is not just the frontline clinicians that are difficult to hire and retain. Hospital executive positions have high turnover. As many as half of nurse executives, and 14 to 18 per cent of chief executive officers, will leave their jobs in a year. Pervasive staffing problems challenge the ability of the hospital to perform its most fundamental functions.

Studies show that there is an association between registered nurse staffing and hospital related mortality, failure to rescue, and higher risk of complications, among other negative patient outcomes. In addition, beds that are not staffed cannot be filled by patients, undermining the admissions process, especially admissions from the emergency department (ED). Nearly half of all hospital emergency departments report being at or over capacity, and the majority of urban hospitals experience time on diversion – when they are closed to incoming ambulances.

The primary reason for going on diversion is a lack of staffed critical care beds. Staffing shortages, overall, are among the top five conditions that lead to ambulance diversion. In addition to ED overcrowding and diversion, about half of hospitals report that staffing shortages contribute to decreased staff satisfaction. Decreased patient satisfaction, reduced numbers of staffed beds, increased length of stay, increased wait times for surgery, as well as cancelled surgeries also follow in the wake of staffing shortages.

Low staff satisfaction is a persistent problem for many hospitals. Hospital-based nurses, for instance, have job dissatisfaction rates that are three to four times higher than the average U.S. worker. Low dissatisfaction rates among nurses is not an American phenomenon, but occurs in other countries where it has been studied, such as Canada, England and Scotland. Yet, the sentiment is not universal. Nurses employed in facilities that have been awarded Magnet Recognition® from the American Nurses Credentialing Center (ANCC) report being more satisfied with their work.

In addition to higher staff satisfaction, Magnet status strengthens nursing recruitment and retention efforts. Independent studies show that patients in Magnet hospitals have shorter lengths of stay, lower mortality rates and higher satisfaction, and benefit from a richer staff mix.

A Global Predicament

As perhaps the most in-demand health care resource across the globe, plenty of nurses are being "insourced" into other countries. The U.S. has long depended on migrating nurses to fill its growing gap between nurse supply and demand. This practice also occurs in other highly developed countries, at the expense of the less developed, where many migrating nurses originate.

Nurses are not the only migrating health care worker. Physicians, pharmacists and lab technicians are on the move as well. The WHO reports that the situation of migrating workers is most desperate in poor countries and continents. Africa, for instance, holds 11 per cent of the world's population, but it hosts 25 per cent of the disease burden, and yet, it employs three per cent of all health care workers. Twenty-five per cent of African-trained doctors work in wealthy Organisation for Economic Co-operation and Development (OECD) countries. In Ghana, 40 physicians graduated in 2004 from the government- financed medical education system, but only two remained in the country. The others left for either the U.S. or U.K. to practice. The shortage of health care workers is exacerbating the devastation wrought by the AIDS crisis in Africa.

According to the WHO, because of the shortage of health care workers at least 1.3 billion people around the world have no access to basic health care services. In response, the WHO is pressing countries across the globe to address the ethical and financial impacts of worker migration, as well as efforts to retain workers within their country of origin. The practice of health care worker importation and exportation is, of course, unsustainable. But, it begs the question: Who will staff the hospital of the future?

Stops and Starts

In the U.S., a poor economy is driving people back to work and providing some optimism for a more robust nursing workforce. New research finds that after a net loss of more than 10,500 nurses in 2004 and 2005, health care gained roughly 18,700 nurses in 2006.

In 2007, the industry added 84,200 nurses despite a drop in real wages. Current projections for the shortage of nurses in the U.S. puts the number at 340,000 by 2020, which is significantly fewer than previous projections of 760,000. An important distinction of the evolving shortage is that the nurses who have stepped forward to help fill the gap are markedly older in their late twenties and early thirties – whereas the number of new entries in their early to mid-twenties is at the lowest level in 40 years.

As the average age of the nurse moves upward, there are implications for hospital design and ergonomics that are needed to support the health and longevity of the nurse on the job. During the first year on the job, the average voluntary turnover rate of new hospital nurses is 27 per cent.

This likely reflects the combination of inadequate educational preparation of the nurse for the realities of practice, as well as longstanding work environment issues that have contributed to low satisfaction rates of hospital-employed nurses. Among these issues are long shifts and persistent fatigue; lack of leadership that empowers nursing staff; unavailability of supportive technologies; and lack of innovation in redesigning and improving the role and workflow of the nurse.

A recent time and motion study to determine how medical-surgical nurses spend their time found that nearly three-quarters of nurses' time was spent on documentation, medication administration and care coordination, but only one-fifth of their time was spent on direct patient care. Further, nurses walked between one mile and five miles every shift in an effort to "hunt and gather" needed supplies or information.

The inordinate amount of time spent on documentation – almost one-third of all of their time – points to the need to examine the role of the nurse and its inherent processes. Few nurses would cite "paperwork," as necessary as it is, as the reason they chose nursing as their profession. A major bottleneck in efforts to add new nurses to the workforce remains a lack of capacity at the educational level. According to data from the American Association of Colleges of Nursing (AACN), enrollment in entry-level baccalaureate nursing programmes increased by almost five per cent from 2006 to 2007.

While this increase represents a positive enrollment trend over the past several years, more than 30,000 qualified applicants were denied entry into baccalaureate nursing programmes in 2007 due primarily to an intensifying shortage of nurse faculty. The gap between supply and demand in the nursing workforce will be difficult to fill without resolution of the crisis in nursing education capacity.

High Touch, High Tech

As patients' needs and health care delivery become ever-more complex, it is difficult for clinicians to keep pace. Hospitalized patients have higher acuity and are more likely to have comorbidities, while hospital stays have shortened. Average length-of-stay for hospitalized patients has declined by 25 per cent since the 1980s.

Since the late 1990s, the Food and Drug Administration (FDA) has approved more than 500,000 new medical devices. At the same time, ever-increasing developments in pharmaceuticals, biologics and genomics are expanding the knowledge demands of practitioners. While many advances in technology help to improve patient outcomes, the sheer volume of technologies and the attendant knowledge required has made health care delivery vastly more complex.

Additionally, new technologies often provide new, sometimes unforeseen, opportunities for error. The impact of this developing complexity weighs heavily on the hospital-based clinician. One way in which the nursing profession has responded is by the creation of the Clinical Nurse Leader™ role. The American Association of Colleges of Nursing (AACN) has developed this new nursing role to better prepare nurses for clinical leadership in all health care settings.

These masters'-prepared nurses are expected to be direct caregivers, managing the care of patients within clinical microsystems. The Clinical Nurse Leader™ certification process ensures that these nurses bring evidencebased practices to care settings and are able to apply quality improvement principles to the measurement, assessment and improvement of patientcare outcomes.

According to the AACN, currently about 60 colleges and universities offer the master's degree programme that prepares the Clinical Nurse Leader.™ Scientific progress, such as new developments in biologics, genomics, robotic preparation and automated distribution, is affecting the level of technologic expertise that the hospital pharmacist must have. In fact, the profession raised the entry-level degree for a pharmacist to a doctorate (Pharm.D) to ensure a better-prepared pharmacist workforce. Many pharmacists who practice in hospitals also complete residency training.

The downside of this higher standard is that it created a roadblock for the entry of new pharmacy students. Indeed, hospitals surveyed by the AHA reported an eight per cent vacancy rate for pharmacists at the end of 2006.

The role of the hospital pharmacist is expected to change as well. Always a valued member of the health care team, the role of the pharmacist is likely to become more visible in patient-centered care delivery as a way to combat the high volume of medication errors that occur in the hospital setting. As hospital pharmacists become more involved in direct patient care, there is a requisite need to accommodate new learning in the education and training of pharmacy students.

There are concerns that hospitals and health systems may not have the capacity to accommodate the growing numbers of pharmacy students who will require this experiential education. The involvement of pharmacists in direct patient care has also resulted in a greater reliance on trained and certified pharmacy technicians, who assist with the preparation and delivery of medications.

A Changing of the Guard

A changing of the guard has been occurring in hospitals over the last several years, a change that is likely to become the standard in hospitals of the future. Hospitalists – physicians who practice primarily hospital-base care – have been increasingly staffing U.S. hospitals. It is estimated that by 2010, 30,000 hospitalists will be staffing U.S. hospitals. As hospitalists are gaining prevalence, the concept is also expanding from general practice and internal medicine to include medical and surgical specialists.

The recent growth of the hospitalist movement in the U.S. can be attributed to a number of factors. Fewer office-based primary care physicians choose to provide hospital-based care. Work hours for residents, who have traditionally provided 24/7 hospital care, have been reduced in recent years. Hospitalists fill these gaps by providing acute care expertise to patients throughout their hospital stay.

Team-Based Care

With staffing shortages still looming in the hospital of the future, hospitals may need to accomplish more with fewer health professionals. Well functioning teams can get more done than any one individual. Teamwork also has a significantly positive impact on the safety of health care delivery. Studies show that well functioning teams make fewer mistakes than do individuals. Acquisition of team skills does not occur by happenstance.

Health professionals must be educated and trained to value and demonstrate desired team behaviours. To that end, knowledge of teamwork components and the competencies required to effectively participate as team members should be introduced early in health care professional education and fostered throughout professional training and continuing education. Further, teamwork skills, knowledge and performance should be incorporated into the oversight and assessment of health professionals and organizations in order to ensure and sustain its widespread adoption.

Both classroom and simulator-based methodologies can be used for team training. In addition to team skills, members of the care-giving team must have the requisite knowledge and skills to effectively care for older adults and the chronically ill. Today, older adults account for 35 per cent of all hospital stays, 26 per cent of all physician visits, and 34 per cent of all prescriptions. Yet, less than one per cent of registered nurses and pharmacists are certified in geriatrics. While more than 7,000 physicians are currently certified in geriatrics, the need is much greater. By 2030, it is estimated that 36,000 geriatricians will be needed to care for the burgeoning population of older adults.

As the number of older adults and patients with one more chronic illness rises, so too, must the competencies of those who provide their care. Hospitals play a key role in fostering the competence of all health care workers in caring for geriatric patients.

Hospitals must also increase the recruitment and retention of geriatric specialists and caregivers. Team-based care models may be expanded and bolstered by the potential payment model advocated by the Medicare Payment Advisory Commission (MedPAC). MedPAC recommends a bundled Medicare payment approach, under which physicians and hospitals receive a fixed payment for a select set of episodes of care. An episode is defined as the hospital stay plus 30 days after discharge.

Today, physicians and hospitals are paid separately under different payment schemes by CMS for hospital-based care. A bundled approach, it is believed, will reduce variation in costs and quality and encourage joint accountability. This concept will be tested by CMS beginning in January 2009 with its Acute Care Episode (ACE) demonstration, which will offer bundled payment for 28 cardiac and nine orthopedic inpatient surgical services in four states.

Among the many expectations for bundled payment is that it will influence physicians and hospitals to closely integrate their services, which will be necessary in order to accept bundled payments.

DESIGN OF THE PHYSICAL ENVIRONMENT

Safe by Design

Though the recent economic downturn and a tightened credit market has slowed hospital construction in the U.S., there has been a remarkable hospital building boom underway fuelled by increasing demand for health care services and increasingly obsolete hospital plants.

In 2007, $35.4 billion in health care construction projects were completed, more than a $10 billion increase from the previous year. Projections foresee the health care industry among the only bright points for construction in the next couple of years. This investment offers the opportunity to remake the hospital — its design, culture and practices – to better meet the needs of patients and families and the aspirations of those that provide their care.

Building more of the same will freeze into place persistent problems with which hospitals must already contend — such as unsafe care, hospitalacquired infection, and worker fatigue – that otherwise could be mitigated through the application of evidence-based design. Several hundred studies have revealed hospital design characteristics that work for improving patient safety and health care outcomes, and providing a supportive environment for hospital staff.

Yet, most new hospitals are not being built "safe by design." New hospitals will increasingly care for more elderly patients. And, as more care moves out to ambulatory and home settings, hospitalized patients will be the sickest and most vulnerable. More than ever, hospitals will need to be designed to safely accommodate these fragile patients.

Prominent threats to patient safety – medication errors, patient falls, and errors made during patient transfers, among them – can be mitigated through evidence-based design. Better lighting and reduced noise levels can help avoid distractions that often lead to caregiver errors in the medication process.

Decentralized nursing stations allow nurses to better see and hear the patients under their care and observe changes in skin colour and breathing, as well as to prevent falls that occur when a patient is unobserved. Rooms that are designed for the patient bed and bathroom entrance to be seen from the hallway also enhance observation. Multiacuity beds that reduce the number of transfers, or "hand-offs," of patients from one unit to another, in turn, reduce the opportunity for errors to occur.

The regulatory infrastructure can stifle design innovations meant to reduce the risk of patient injury.

Though multi-acuity beds that allow a patient to remain in the same bed while their care level is stepped down from critical care to medical-surgical nursing may make sense, in some states they do not meet state licensure stipulations regarding patient bed designations and thereby are disqualified for reimbursement. Single-patient rooms may have the single most important impact on patient safety. In addition to enhancing patient privacy, allowing for confidential discussions and accommodating family members, single rooms help protect patients' health. Spread of infection is a daily risk in every of hospital. When patients are isolated from one another, there are fewer chances for microbes to be spread. In addition to patient-to-patient spread, caregiverto- patient spread is common.

Well-placed sinks and alcohol gel dispensers can prompt caregivers to wash their hands, which is an essential part of any infection control programme. Single rooms further improve the rate of hand-washing when crossing the barriers between patient rooms prompts caregivers to wash their hands. Whereas, in a double patient room, the transition from one patient to the next is quick and barrier-free; too little time to stop and think about hand-washing. Single rooms also allow for better air quality management and can be more thoroughly decontaminated between occupancies.

Flat World Phenomena

Infection control, always a high priority for any hospital, becomes paramount in the face of a potential global epidemic. Emergency preparedness is a key priority to be addressed in the design of the hospital of the future.

In today's ever-flattening world, individuals are more globalized – they travel more, both virtually and in person. The supply chain is also more globalized and could easily be disrupted by a global epidemic: "...when the world is flattening – when some 80 per cent of the raw materials that go into pharmaceutical drugs sold in America come from overseas suppliers, and when the rubber that keeps surgical masks tight on your face comes through a just-in-time supply chain that starts in Indonesia or Africa, stretches through Europe, and then skips over to America – our ability to cope with any pandemic would be sharply reduced." Thanks to the ubiquity of airline travel, an infectious disease can move quickly in a flat world. Once SARS appeared in rural China, it spread to five countries within 24 hours.

In a matter of months, it had spread to 30 countries on six continents. With the SARS epidemic, hospitals that were sought for care became the vectors for SARS transmission. Open bay intensive care units (ICUs), public waiting areas, and emergency departments all became central stations for contracting SARS. Tuberculosis has also been known to be similarly spread.

The good news is that hospitals can be designed to mitigate these risks. The transformation of the physical environment of care must also take into consideration future needs such as achieving surge capacity in response to disaster.

Standardized Flexibility

- Standardization reduces complexity, which is important when flexibility is needed, as is the case for increasing surge capacity. Importantly, standardization is a key strategy in human factors design as a means to reduce the risk of error and improve quality. Human factors design focuses on improving the human-system interface by designing better systems and processes. For hospitals, standardization of patient rooms, treatment rooms, equipment and care processes, reduces reliance on short-term memory. In room design, standardizing details such as the location of bed controls, light switches, and even, which cupboards store latex gloves, for instance, are important considerations for optimizing the human-system interface. The lengthy cycle of design and construction is often overtaken by the rapid cycle of innovation in medicine and technology. As a result, some buildings are partially obsolete when they open, and nearly every health care structure will be obsolete in some way before it has completed its useful life. Design for flexibility is a way to reduce the inconvenience and cost of these inevitable disruptions. *Master planning strategies:* Every design should have planned zones for future growth. These can appear as a dotted line on the site plan, or may be developed as constructed but unoccupied shell space, or as structural capacity to allow for future vertical additions to a building.
- *Loose-fit design:* Many designs make an effort to design precisely to the absolute minimum square footage justified by the programme of space requirements, yet such designs are the first to reveal difficulties when new programmes appear, or existing programmes grow or shrink. The concept of loose-fit is to design with larger spaces that can be used for more than the minimum function originally proposed, and to arrange them in departments or groupings that allow for future adjustments.
- *Adaptable flexibility:* Spaces can be designed to adapt to multiple uses. An example is a patient room that can be adapted for the purpose of simple procedures such as a line insertion. The different

function can be accommodated by simply adapting the space because it has been planned to serve a range of possibilities.

- *Convertible flexibility:* Another type of flexibility is when, with relatively low effort, time, and/or cost, a space can be converted to another use. Examples of this type of flexibility include a storage space with a knockout panel in the slab to allow for a future elevator, or a patient room with plumbing, gasses, and electrical systems in the wall for future conversion to critical care.
- *Robust utilities:* In order to offer flexibility in design, the utility and communication infrastructure of a health care facility should be capable of expansion and upgrade. Availability of utility and network capacity simplifies and dramatically reduces the cost of future projects.
- *Plug-and-play infrastructure:* Just as all the utilities of the city are uninterrupted when one property undergoes a construction or demolition project, a hospital should be designed so that the utility and primary horizontal and vertical circulation infrastructure remains in service while departments, wings, or entire buildings are added or removed.

Place of Work

In addition to protecting patients, hospital design is integral to protecting hospital workers and enhancing the work they do. About one-third of a nurse's time on shift is spent walking. Not only is this time spent walking between the centralized nursing station and patient rooms, but on hunting and gathering various supplies.

Decentralizing nursing stations and supplies – bringing both closer to the patients – would reduce wasted time and fatigue. Other physical stressors include noise, that when reduced results in less fatigue and reduced risk of error. A great deal of heavy lifting, turning, and transporting patients goes on in hospitals that could be alleviated by proper hoists and other ergonomic technologies. Involving staff in the design process is essential for creating a physical environment that improves work flow.

In the future, the application of design improvements to time-consuming nursing tasks, such as medication administration and documentation, may yield new gains in efficiency. As pharmacists increasingly counsel patients on drugs and therapeutic regimens, the physical environment of the pharmacy must be made to accommodate these confidential discussions.

New design concepts have been shown to give hospital clinical staff more time to spend with patients, while also allowing the hospital to expand its capacity to treat patients. Designing a hospital with safety in mind helps to create a safety culture.

Involving patients and families, in addition to staff, in the design of the physical environment also helps to assure the patientcenteredness of the organizational culture.

The culture of the workplace can be transformed by the physical demonstration that the organization embraces patient and staff safety, and collegial health care delivery.

Being Green

Global climate change and harm wrought from chemical contamination are no longer speculative. In congruence with their mission, hospitals in the future must be healthy places to be in and live near. In 1996, the Environmental Protection Agency (EPA) declared medical waste incineration to be the greatest source of dioxin contamination in the atmosphere. At that time, there were 5,000 medical waste incinerators. Today there are fewer than 100 still in operation.

That momentum needs to continue and be broadened to include the elimination of toxic materials used inside the hospital. The chemical compound polyvinyl chloride (PVC) is ubiquitous in the hospital environment. It is used in I.V. and blood bags, plastic tubing and an array of other medical supplies.

When PVCbased products, such as nasogastric tubes, are used invasively, they can leach toxic chemicals that enter the body. One of these chemicals has proven to be a reproductive toxicant, which led the National Toxicology Programme to declare that infants in hospitals are at risk from this chemical. PVC, which is also commonly used in hospital building materials, emits toxins into the air, putting patients and staff at risk.

Interior exposure to PVC has been definitively linked to asthma. With the prevalence of PVC exposure, as well as exposure to other noxious chemicals such as cleaning agents and pesticides, it is no wonder that poor air quality is the most frequent cause of work-related asthma in health care workers. Hospitals are huge consumers of energy – natural gas and electricity — second only to the food-service industry in energy consumption. The costs of such energy consumption will increasingly comprise an unaffordable portion of the hospital budget.

These costs plus growing concern over global warming are influencing hospitals to use cleaner, more efficient sources of energy and to reduce their global footprint. Accordingly, hospitals will need to use fewer resources and produce less waste.

One hundred U.S. hospitals are finding it easier to be green by piloting the *Green Guide for Health Care (GGHC)*, standards modeled on those of the U.S. Green Building Council's Leadership in Energy and Environmental Design (LEED), in their construction projects. The GGHC standards actually exceed LEED standards and align environmental health considerations with health system priorities.

The GGHC has received strong endorsement – Kaiser Permanente has committed to using it for building projects across its system, and the City of Boston is recommending it to city hospitals that are embarking on expansion plans. A healthy hospital environment also extends to the food that is served in that environment. Food that is served in hospitals should promote and not undermine health.

Large health care systems, such as Kaiser Permanente and Catholic Health care West, have led the way in implementing policies that require healthy food choices for patients and also support sustainable farming practices – food production that is local, humane and environmentally protective.

6

Nurses in Hospital Planning, Working with Administration and Management

Good nurses are professionals who strive to make a positive impact in their organizations. Some are able to make this impact by working in planning with hospital administrators. The minority nurse who works in planning is in a pivotal role for making sure patients are safe, says Evelina Echols-Sutton, BSN, RN, nursing director of Women and Children's Services at Methodist Charlton Medical Center in Dallas, Texas. These professionals often have leadership titles, such as nurse manager or nurse director. Or they may be in specialty roles, such as nurse statistician and nursing informatics, she says. But one common theme is that they are called on to share ideas with their organization's leadership.

"They are in those key meetings where decisions are made on the policies that we adopt, the equipment that we eventually bring in to our facility, and the streamlined workflows that will make sure our patients and family are safe," says Glenda Totten, RN, MSN, CNS, director of nursing services at Kaiser Permanente Los Angeles Medical Center in California.

On an average workday, a nurse who works in planning may interact with the director of pharmacy, information technology, environmental services, human resources, risk management, and legal departments, says Echols-Sutton. "My typical day is probably about four hours of meetings, four hours of office work, and then four hours of follow-up on all these activities."

"Meetings are also a constant variable in my day," says Sylvia Williams, RN, MSN, director of education and inpatient nursing services at La Rabida Children's Hospital in Chicago, Illinois. "They range from brainstorming meetings on quality initiatives to troubleshooting staffing concerns. On average, I would say I am in meetings a good five to six hours per day. They are important to keep morale high and ensure everyone works together harmoniously."

Kanoe Allen, RN, MSN-CNS, PHN, ONC, is chief nursing officer at Hoag Orthopedic Institute in Irvine, California. She says that nurses who work in planning have to juggle meetings with idea generation. "One of the challenges is carving out time to sit quietly and think through the issues and to have time to develop solutions," says Allen.

Unsurprisingly, nurse leaders are better compensated for their efforts. The median pay for a nurse manager is $77,988, while it's only $55,447 for a registered nurse, according to Payscale.com. Hospitals in turn get someone who engages in positive relationships within nursing, and with managers, supervisors, staff nurses, and executive leaders, says Totten. "It takes all that to make it work and have a world-class facility."

MANAGING INSIDE AND OUT

In addition to working with leadership, minority nurses in hospital planning also have to help manage their organizations' external pressures, says Totten. There are numerous outside factors to consider, such as working to meet the standards established by the Joint Commission. As an example, Totten regularly conferences with a stroke performance improvement committee to help her facility earn a comprehensive designation from the Joint Commission.

"It's ensuring that for any [stroke] patient that goes to our emergency room, or any that are inpatients, we react immediately. We get the neurology resident in there and get the team in there within seconds," she says.

Totten also works on a nursing quality improvement committee to assess nurse sensitive measures, such as interventions that help prevent falls in the hospital. Her teams are responsible for coming up with tools to communicate with nurses so that they are quickly informed about any relevant changes within the medical facility. "We plan for our 1,200 or so nurses to make sure that everyone, including the per diem nurses, know what's coming, what's changing, how they can get more education, and the kinds of tools they need so that they're up-to-date with the changes," explains Totten. Another planning team is responsible for providing constructive criticism to nurses on meeting patients. This involves communicating the best ways to exhibit caring behaviors, such as pulling up a chair and sitting eyeball to eyeball with those they serve, says Totten.

"It's evidence-based and proven that you don't want to stand over [patients]. You want to be as close to them as possible," she notes.

"We're trying to standardize how we greet our patients when they come in on admission and also while they're here." These issues are important because of the new value-based purchasing environment, says Shawana Burnette, OB-RNC, MSN, CLNC, a nurse manager in High Risk Post Partum and High Risk OB at Carolinas Medical Center in Charlotte, North Carolina.

A portion of reimbursements received from the Centers for Medicare and Medicaid Services will be based on the patient's value perception of the care they receive, she explains. This means nurses in planning have to encourage their teams to not only help the patient heal, but to also have a good bedside manner. Another area where nurses who work in planning are called on to help is to find ways to improve infection rates. The Centers for Disease Control and Prevention as well as the Institute for Healthcare Improvement review these rates, and of course, the goal is to have them as low as possible, says Totten. "You have to plan how you can show that you have a stellar place."

Medical centers also compete with other health care centers in the community. "The consumer is more astute nowadays, and they are open to shop for the best medical facility, best health care facility, and the best insurance," she notes. This means nurses who work in planning often need to represent their medical centers to the community. "We have a foundation that does fundraising. In order to help them, I have to go out and speak," says Echols-Sutton. "You want to talk to those that you serve, and find out what's important to them."

IMPROVING SOFT SKILLS, LEVERAGING CLINICAL SKILLS

First, health care is a highly regulated industry. Second, reimbursements are based upon the customers' perceptions of "soft" skills, explains Allen. "Putting the two together is a change for this industry." Fortunately, nurses are usually well-prepared. "Nurses, by their calling, have a set of innate behaviors of putting people and solutions to the front," says Allen. "It is a team spirit, not an individual-only spirit. That is key to the success of multidisciplinary patient care." People come to nursing with a big heart and a desire to help others, and it serves them well in collaborative environments where they have to work together to find the solutions, she adds.

Allen notes that being successful in nurse planning requires emotional intelligence, meaning the ability to understand and have a sense of another person's views. To achieve success in planning means being a team player, using that emotional intelligence to understand the interplay between various personalities and departments, and working in a collaborative manner to solve regulatory and other issues, she says.

Minority nurses who work in planning can also help bridge multicultural gaps. Multicultural environments are a challenge to blend and the goal is to bring out the best attributes, says Allen. "We serve patients from many backgrounds and having a diverse staff allows us to better anticipate and understand their cultural needs," notes Williams.

Soft skills are necessary in higher levels of planning, but practical experience is also important, explains Totten. "One thing you can never take away from a nurse is her clinical skills. It's handy when you're working in a clinical setting. The more you move up in your career, [the more] those clinical skills are key." It all comes down to ensuring that staff members have the correct resources to care for patients, says Allen. Providing the right resources allows the staff to provide strong patient care. "Staff who do not have to worry about resources and administration support provide great customer service," she adds.

The Career Path

Minority nurses who want to work with hospital administrators, or who want to be in administration themselves, have multiple options. "The best thing about the profession of nursing is you can pretty much take any path. You can be in a clinical track and still move up to administration. There is also the education track, nurse practitioner track, and advanced practice nursing," says Totten. "All these elements can secure you a good position in administration."

Totten's own background is as a clinical nurse specialist, but she emphasizes there are many ways to advance. As a first step, Burnette suggests becoming a bachelor's-prepared nurse. "They have the four-year preparation that includes handling more professional issues and critical thinking," she explains. "The classes prepare you to be in a leadership role."

But you should also have your sights set on earning a master's degree. "Years of experience on the nursing unit are critical, but I would strongly recommend to anyone that is interested in this path to pursue an advanced degree in nursing," says Williams. "Nurses who work in planning need knowledge-based skills like budgeting and financials, experience you don't necessarily receive on the floor," she continues. The more educated you are regarding the area you're going in, the more prepared you will be.

Mentoring

Another important means for having a successful career in hospital planning is to find a mentor who can show you the ropes in a real life environment, notes Williams. "There are many ups and downs in nursing. There are plenty of wonderful days, and there are days in which nothing seems to go right. Being able to balance the good with the bad is essential to having a long career in nursing," argues Williams. A good mentor can instill these lessons to their mentees and help them find their way, she adds.

Mentoring is intended to help nurses develop their skills and grow within the nursing profession. "The mentor accomplishes this by sharing their years of experiences—warts and all—to help them see nursing in its true light," explains Williams.

Mentoring also helps a person explore who they are and how they can achieve more in their career, says Allen. In some cases, it opens doors for opportunity as well. "I have had a mentor who challenges my thoughts and plans, refocuses me when I am at a loss and then cheers me on," she continues.

Having a mentor can also help nurses develop critical work skills, such as priority setting, stress management, people management, and good communication, says Echols-Sutton. She hasn't had an "official" mentor, but she has had role models she patterned herself after. Other nurses who aren't in employee-sponsored mentor programs can do the same, she notes.

"I didn't have just one person. I tried to learn from everybody, including coworkers, bosses, and even people out in the community," says Echols-Sutton. "They were available for me to pick their brains." Burnette advises nurses to find mentors who are not necessarily in their departments. If you talk to someone who works in another area of the hospital, they can give you a more global view of your organization. It's important to surround yourself with people who have different perspectives but who are committed to achieving the same goal of providing patients with the best possible health care, she adds. Whether a nurse joins a formal preceptor program or starts an informal mentoring friendship, anyone who wants to work in planning should reach out to a health care professional with more experience to help them along, argues Totten. "It's not just enough to sit in your position."

WORKING WITH ADMINISTRATION

Hospital administrators face many challenges from staffing to budgeting, and it is impossible to have a "go alone" mindset, says Williams. That's why nurses who are in planning are a vital part of the team. Nurses who work with hospital administration report that their careers are fulfilling, and they have a large say in improving their hospitals.

"When you're working in planning, you're able to communicate with all the various staff as well as patients. It gives you a love for the ways you can improve the care that's delivered to patients," says Williams. "That's where you can make the biggest impact."

HOSPITAL, HEALTH CARE AND NURSING

A hospital is an institution for health care providing patient treatment by specialized staff and equipment, and often, but not always providing for longer-term patient stays.

Today, hospitals usually are funded by the public sector, by health organizations, (for profit or nonprofit), health insurance companies or charities, including by direct charitable donations. In history, however, hospitals often were founded and funded by religious orders or charitable individuals and leaders. Similarly, modern-day hospitals are largely staffed by professional physicians, surgeons, and nurses, whereas in history, this work usually was performed by the founding religious orders or by volunteers.

Etymology

During the Middle Ages the hospital could serve other functions, such as almshouse for the poor, hostel for pilgrims, or hospital school. The name comes from Latin *hospes* (host), which also is the root for the English words *hospice*, *hotel*, *hostel*, and *hospitality*. The modern word *hotel* derives from the French word *hostel*, which featured a silent, eventually removed from the word to leave a circumflex on modern French *hotel.* The word also is related to the German word 'Spital'.

Grammar of the word differs slightly depending on the dialect. In the U.S., *hospital* usually requires an article; in Britain and elsewhere, the word normally is used without an article when it is the object of a preposition and when referring to a patient ("in/to the hospital" vs. "in/ to hospital"); in Canada, both uses are found.

Types

Some patients go to a hospital just for diagnosis, treatment, or therapy and then leave ('outpatients') without staying overnight; while others are 'admitted' and stay overnight or for several weeks or months ('inpatients'). Hospitals usually are distinguished from other types of medical facilities by their ability to admit and care for inpatients and the others often are described as a clinic.

General

The best-known type of hospital is the general hospital, which is set up to deal with many kinds of disease and injury, and typically has an emergency department to deal with immediate and urgent threats to health. A general hospital typically is the major health care facility in its region, with large numbers of beds for intensive care and long-term care; and specialized facilities for surgery, plastic surgery, childbirth, bioassay laboratories, and so forth. Larger cities may have many several hospitals of varying sizes and facilities. Some hospitals, especially in the United States, have their own ambulance service.

Specialized

Types of specialized hospitals include trauma centres, rehabilitation hospitals, children's hospitals, seniors' (geriatric) hospitals, and hospitals for dealing with specific medical needs such as psychiatric problems, certain disease categories, and so forth.

A hospital may be a single building or a number of buildings on a campus. Many hospitals with pre-twentieth-century origins began as one building and evolved into campuses. Some hospitals are affiliated with universities for medical research and the training of medical personnel such as physicians and nurses, often called teaching hospitals. Worldwide, most hospitals are run on a nonprofit basis by governments or charities. Within the United States, most hospitals are nonprofit.

Teaching

A teaching hospital combines assistance to patients with teaching to medical students and nurses and often is linked to a medical school or nursing school. Some of these are associated with universities

Clinics

A medical facility smaller than a hospital is generally called a clinic, and often is run by a government agency for health services or a private partnership of physicians (in nations where private practice is allowed). Clinics generally provide only outpatient services.

Departments

Hospitals vary widely in the services they offer and therefore, in the departments they have. They may have acute services such as an emergency department or specialist trauma centre, burn unit, surgery, or urgent care. These may then be backed up by more specialist units such as cardiology or coronary care unit, intensive care unit, neurology, cancer centre, and obstetrics and gynecology.

Some hospitals will have outpatient departments and some will have chronic treatment units such as behavioural health services, dentistry, dermatology, psychiatric ward, rehabilitation services, and physical therapy.

Common support units include a dispensary or pharmacy, pathology, and radiology, and on the non-medical side, there often are medical records departments and/or release of information department.

ACUTE ASSESSMENT UNIT

An acute assessment unit, or acute admissions unit, (AAU) is a short-stay department in UK hospitals that is sometimes part of the emergency department, although a separate department. The AAU acts as a gateway between a patient's general practitioner, the emergency department, and the wards of the hospital. The AAU helps the emergency department produce a healthy turnaround for patients, helping with the four-hour waiting rule.

An AAU is usually made up of several bays and has a small number of side-rooms and treatment rooms. They are fully equipped with emergency medical treatment facilities including defibrilators and resuscitation equipment.

Patients

From the emergency department, patients can be moved to AAU where they will undergo further tests and stabilisation before they are transferred to the relevant ward or sent home. Also, patients can be admitted straight to AAU from their general practitioner if he or she believes the patient needs hospital treatment. A patient's stay in the unit is limited, usually no more than 48 hours.

The AAU deals with admissions only, patients will never be transferred from a ward to the AAU. Surgical Procedures are not carried out in the unit either; these are referred on to the relevant theatre such as cardiothoracics and general surgery.

Staff

Senior staff in an AAU include a consultant in general medicine, emergency medicine, or critical care. Often a registrar in general medicine, and a ward sister or a charge nurse have roles in the unit. A number of staff nurses work alongside the senior staff to provide care to patients in the unit. Although AAU has its own staff trained to deal with patients and provide care, members of staff from other departments in the hospital are needed in AAU to assess patients and provide further diagnosis. Typical examples of staff who may be needed in AAU are general surgeons, cardiothoracic surgeons, cardiologists, and a psychiatric liaison nurse.

Alternative Names for the Department

Different hospitals use different names for the department - common names for this department are:

- Acute Assessment Unit
- Acute Admissions Unit
- Clinical Decision Unit (CDU)
- Medical Assessment Unit (MAU)
- Multi speciality Assessment Area (MSAA)
- Medical Receiving Unit (MRU)
- Emergency Receiving Unit (ERU)

CORONARY CARE UNIT

A coronary care unit (CCU) is a hospital ward specialized in the care of patients with heart attacks, unstable angina and (in practice) various other cardiac conditions that require continuous monitoring and treatment.

Characteristics

The main feature of coronary care is the availability of telemetry or the continuous monitoring of the cardiac rhythm by electrocardiography. This allows early intervention with medication, cardioversion or defibrillation, improving the prognosis.

As arrhythmias are relatively common in this group, patients with myocardial infarction or unstable angina are routinely admitted to the coronary care unit. For other indications, such as atrial fibrillation, a specific indication is generally necessary, while for others, such as heart block, coronary care unit admission is standard.

Local Differences

In the United States, coronary care units are usually subsets of intensive care units (ICU) dedicated to the care of critically ill cardiac patients. These units are usually present in hospitals that routine engage in cardiothoracic surgery. Invasive monitoring such as with pulmonary artery catheters is common, as are supportive modalities such as mechanical ventilation and intra-aortic balloon pumps (IABP).

Certain hospitals, such as Johns Hopkins, maintain mixed units consisting of both Acute care units for the critically ill, and intermediate care units for patients who are not critical.

Acute Coronary Care

Acute coronary care units (ACCU), also called "critical coronary care units" (CCCU) is equivalent to intensive care in the level of service provided. Patients with acute myocardial infarction, cardiogenic shock, or post-operative "open-heart" patients commonly abide here.

Subacute Coronary Care

Subacute coronary care units (SCCU), also called Progressive care units (PCU), Intermediate coronary care units (ICCU), or stepdown units, and provide a level of care intermediate to that of the intensive care unit and that of the general medical floor. These units typically serve patients who require cardiac telemetry such as those with unstable angina.

Coronary care units developed in the 1960s when it became clear that close monitoring by specially trained staff, cardiopulmonary resuscitation and medical measures could reduce the mortality from complications of cardiovascular disease. The first description of a CCU was given in 1961 to the British Thoracic Society, and early CCUs were located in Sydney, Kansas City and Philadelphia. Studies published in 1967 revealed that those observed in a coronary care setting had consistently better outcomes. The first coronary care unit was opened at Bethany Medical Centre in Kansas City, Kansas by Dr. Hugh Day, and he coined the term. Bethany Medical Centre is also where the first "crash carts" were developed.

EMERGENCY DEPARTMENT

The Emergency Department (ED), sometimes termed Accident & Emergency (A&E), Emergency Room (ER), Emergency Ward (EW), or Casualty Department is a hospital or primary care department that provides initial treatment to patients with a broad spectrum of illnesses and injuries, some of which may be life-threatening and require immediate attention. In some countries, Emergency Departments have become important entry points for those without other means of access to medical care. Staff teams treat emergency patients and provide support to family members. The emergency departments of most hospitals operate around the clock, although staffing levels attempt to mirror patient volume, which in most ED's finds its nadir between 2:00 am and 6:00 am. Most patients seek the Emergency Department in the afternoon and evening hours, and staffing mirrors this phenomenon.

History

The first specialized trauma care centre in the world was opened in 1911 in the United States at the University of Louisville Hospital in Louisville, Kentucky, and was developed by surgeon Arnold Griswold during the 1930s. Griswold also equipped police and fire vehicles with medical supplies and trained officers to give emergency care while en route to the hospital.

Department Layout

A typical emergency department has several different areas, each specialized for patients with particular severities or types of illness.

In the *triage* area, patients are seen by an RN or LPN, who completes a preliminary evaluation, before they are transferred to another area of the ED or a different department in the hospital. One body of expertise that seems particularly applicable to emergency medicine services is Operations Management. Operations management utilizes a systems approach to the provision of a service, including the definition of the particular characteristics of a service (such as the service package, the service process, and the virtual value chain embedded in that service), structured planning for service quality, appropriate service metrics, selected management tools, and consideration of strategies for interdisciplinary collaboration, as well as cultural change. The*resuscitation* area is a key ultimately, the value of an operations management approach to management of the ED is explicit consideration of all salient elements of the service process in a systematic manner.

In doing so, it is important to link clearly the service function to the institutions mission/strategic plan, as well as the expectations and needs of ED patients who are served there. They are sent to the *minors* area. Such patients may still have been found to have significant problems, including fractures, dislocations, and lacerations requiring suturing.

Asplin (A Conceptual Model of Emergency Department Crowding. Ann Emerg Med. 2003; 42:173-180), describes a three-phase "input – throughput – output" model of emergency services. This model is applicable to the challenge and solutions to the problem of ED overcrowding that has occurred in many communities in the US.

The information paper includes the following sections:

Some departments employ a *play therapist* whose job is to put children at ease to reduce the anxiety caused by visiting the emergency department, as well as provide distraction therapy for simple procedures.

Many hospitals have a separate area for evaluation of psychiatric problems. These are often staffed by psychiatrists and mental health nurses and social workers. There is typically at least one room for people who are actively a risk to themselves or others (e.g. suicidal).

Intangibility: Services are not manufactured according to precise standards, nor can they be stored. How consumers perceive services is very subjective, since they are a performance rather than a tangible good. Variability: Consistent service delivery is very difficult, particularly in fields such as medicine, due to the high labour contribution of the service along with the variation between clinicians. Inseparability: Service quality is extremely difficult to control since it is produced and consumed at the same time. There is no opportunity to measure or inspect the service prior to actually delivering it. Additionally, the consumer (patient) significantly impacts the quality of the service provided. For example, the description of a patient's symptoms can significantly affect the outcome of the visit. The better the description, the more likely a better outcome.

Signage

A hospital with an emergency department usually has prominent signage reading *Emergency* or *Accident and Emergency* (often in white text on a red background) and an arrow to indicate where patients should proceed. Some American states closely regulate the design and content of such signs and require wording such as "Comprehensive Emergency Medical Service" and "Physician On Duty", to prevent persons in need of critical care from presenting to facilities that are not fully equipped and staffed.

Nomenclature

In Australia and Canada, the department is usually referred to as the *Emergency Department* or *Emerg.*

In the United Kingdom, New Zealand, Hong Kong, Singapore, and Ireland specifically, the department is known as *A&E* (Accident & Emergency). In response to the number of 'minor' injuries that are often presented within the department, some hospitals now choose to only use the term *ED* (Emergency Department) in order to emphasise urgent cases only. Despite this, all road signs to the department throughout the UK read *A&E*, and this remains unchanged. Most teaching hospitals and district general hospitals (DGHs) have an A&E department. The largest such department in the UK is in the city of Leicester (Leicester Royal Infirmary). The term *Casualty*, which preceded A&E in the UK (and is still at times informally used to denote the emergency department of a hospital) is no longer considered appropriate by emergency medical staff in the United Kingdom and Ireland, for similar aforementioned reasons.

In the United States an emergency department is often referred to by both laypeople and medical professionals as an *emergency room* or an "ER." [Medical professionals occasionally call it whatever its name is within their specific hospitals, or simply "emergency."] The term "emergency room" is based on historic usage and is a misnomer today, for a modern hospital's emergency facilities do not consist of only a single room. The ER interacts with every other department in the hospital and often represents a significant percentage of the hospital's work load and finances.

During the 1990s, an effort began to change to the more accurate term *emergency department* (ED), which is a term increasingly used by members of the specialty internationally. The updated name has not yet caught on to the mainstream American public, perhaps due in part to the popularity of the TV show *ER*, and the heavy marketing of the abbreviation "ED" for erectile dysfunction by pharmaceutical companies. However, the term does have wide circulation among emergency medicine staff. Individual hospitals may also refer to the department by different names, such as emergency ward, emergency centre, emergency unit, etc.

Leading journals, including the Annals of Emergency Medicine, published by the American College of Emergency Physicians, and the Emergency Medicine Journal (emj) of the British Association for Emergency Medicine (BAEM), consistently use the term *emergency department*.

In some countries, including the United States, Europe and Canada, a smaller facility that may provide assistance in medical emergencies is known as a clinic. Larger communities often have walk-in clinics where people with medical problems that would not be considered serious enough to warrant an emergency department visit can be seen. These clinics often do not operate on a 24 hour basis.

The term "urgency" instead of "emergency" is used in some Latin American countries. Emergency departments are known as *"servicios de urgencia"* and they function in a similar fashion to European emergency departments.

United States

Many U.S. emergency rooms are exceedingly busy. A survey of New York area doctors in February 2007 found that injuries and even deaths have been caused by excessive waits for hospital beds by ER patients. A 2005 patient survey found an average ER wait time from 2.3 hours in Iowa to 5.0 hours in Arizona.

One inspection of Los Angeles area hospitals by Congressional staff found the ERs operating at an average of 116% of capacity (meaning there were more patients than available treatment spaces) with insufficient beds to accommodate victims of a terrorist attack the size of the 2004 Madrid train bombings. Three of the five Level I trauma centres were on "diversion", meaning ambulances with all but the most severely injured patients were being directed elsewhere because the ER could not safely accommodate any more patients. This controversial practice was banned in Massachusetts (except for major incidents, such as a fire in the ER), effective January 1, 2009; in response, hospitals have devoted more staff to the ER at peak times and moved some elective procedures to non-peak times.

United Kingdom

All A&E departments throughout the United Kingdom are financed and managed by the NHS of each constituent country (England, Scotland, Wales and Northern Ireland). As with most other NHS services, emergency care is provided to all, both resident citizens and those not ordinarily resident in the UK, free at the point of need and regardless of any ability to pay.

Historically, waits for assessment in A&E were very long in some areas of the UK. In October 2002, the Department of Health introduced a four-hour target in emergency departments that required departments to assess and treat patients within four hours of arrival, with referral and assessment by other departments if deemed necessary. Present policy is that 98% of all patient cases do not "breach" this four-hour wait.

The 4-hour target triggered the introduction of the acute assessment unit (also known as the medical assessment unit), which works alongside the emergency department but is outside it for statistical purposes in the bed management cycle. It is claimed that though A&E targets have resulted in significant improvements in completion times, the current target would not have been possible without some form of patient re-designation or re-labelling taking place, so true improvements are somewhat less than headline figures might suggest and it is doubtful that a single target (fitting all A&E and related services) is sustainable.

Patient Experience

If the patient's service expectation is not met, there are ways to remedy this shortcoming. Service recovery is an effective tool to prevent patient defection, but it is necessary to have a well crafted plan in place before the actual event occurs. Patient retention can have a significant financial impact.

Patients are becoming more sophisticated and the healthcare industry must take notice of this. Other sectors of the economy are providing an ever higher quality of service and are raising consumers' expectations along with it. If budget motels, low cost airlines and quick auto lube outlets can produce consistently high quality service encounters, patients will only come to expect that much and more from high-tech and high-cost medical encounters.

CRITICAL CONDITIONS HANDLED

Cardiac Arrest

Cardiac arrest may occur in the ED/A&E or a patient may be transported by ambulance to the emergency department already in this state. Treatment is basic life support and advanced life support as taught in advanced life support and advanced cardiac life support courses. This is an immediately life-threatening condition which requires immediate action in salvageable cases.

Heart Attack

Patients arriving to the emergency department with a myocardial infarction (heart attack) are likely to be triaged to the resuscitation area. They will receive oxygen and monitoring and have an early ECG; aspirin will be given if not contraindicated or not already administered by the ambulance team; morphine or diamorphine will be given for pain; sub lingual (under the tongue) or buccal (between cheek and upper gum) glyceryl trinitrate [nitroglycerin] (GTN or NTG) will be given, unless contraindicated by the presence of other drugs, such as drugs that treat erectile dysfunction.

An ECG that reveals ST segment elevation or new left bundle branch block suggests complete blockage of one of the main coronary arteries. These patients require immediate reperfusion (re-opening) of the occluded vessel. This can be achieved in two ways: [thrombolysis] (clot-busting medication) or percutaneous transluminal coronary angioplasty (PTCA). Both of these are effective in reducing significantly the mortality of myocardial infarction. Many centres are now moving to the use of PTCA as it is somewhat more effective than thrombolysis if it can be administered early. This may involve transfer to a nearby facility with facilities for angioplasty.

Trauma

Major trauma, the term for patients with multiple injuries, often from a road traffic accident or a fall, is treated by a trauma team who have been trained using the principles taught in the internationally recognized Advanced Trauma Life Support (ATLS) course of the American College of Surgeons. Some other international training bodies have started to run similar courses based on the same principles.

The services that are provided in an emergency department can range from simple x-rays and the setting of broken bones to those of a full-scale trauma centre. A patient's chance of survival is greatly improved if the patient receives definitive treatment (i.e. surgery or reperfusion) within one hour of an accident (such as a car accident) or onset of acute illness (such as a heart attack). This critical time frame is commonly known as the "golden hour."

Some emergency departments in smaller hospitals are located near a helipad which is used by helicopters to transport a patient to a trauma centre. This inter-hospital transfer is often done when a patient requires advanced medical care unavailable at the local facility. In such cases the emergency department can only stabilize the patient for transport.dr jawed

Mental Illness

Some patients arrive at an emergency department for a complaint of mental illness. In many jurisdictions (including many U.S. states), patients who appear to be mentally ill and to present a danger to themselves or others may be brought against their will to an emergency department by law enforcement officers for psychiatric examination. The emergency department conducts medical clearance rather and treats acute behavioural disorders. From the emergency department, patients with significant mentally illness may be transferred to a psychiatric unit (in many cases involuntarily).

Asthma and COPD

Acute exacerbations of chronic respiratory diseases, mainly asthma and chronic obstructive pulmonary disease (COPD), are assessed as emergencies and treated with oxygen therapy, bronchodilators, steroids or theophylline, have an urgent chest X-ray and arterial blood gases and are referred for intensive care if necessary. Non invasive ventilation in the ED has reduced the requirement for intubation in many cases of severe exacerbations of COPD.

Special Facilities, Training, and Equipment

An ED requires different equipment and different approaches than most other hospital divisions. Patients frequently arrive with unstable conditions, and so must be treated quickly. They may be unconscious, and information such as their medical history, allergies, and blood type may be unavailable. ED staff are trained to work quickly and effectively even with minimal information.

ED staff must also interact efficiently with pre-hospital care providers such as EMTs, paramedics, and others who are occasionally based in an ED. The pre-hospital providers may use equipment unfamiliar to the average physician, but ED physicians must be expert in using (and safely removing) specialized equipment, since devices such as Military Anti-Shock Trousers ("MAST") and traction splints require special procedures. Among other reasons, given that they must be able to handle specialized equipment, physicians can now specialize in emergency medicine, and EDs employ many such specialists.

ED staff have much in common with ambulance and fire crews, combat medics, search and rescue teams, and disaster response teams. Often, joint training and practice drills are organized to improve the coordination of this complex response system. Busy EDs exchange a great deal of equipment with ambulance crews, and both must provide for replacing, returning, or reimbursing for costly items.

Cardiac arrest and major trauma are relatively common in EDs, so defibrillators, automatic ventilation and CPR machines, and bleeding control dressings are used heavily. Survival in such cases is greatly enhanced by shortening the wait for key interventions, and in recent years some of this specialized equipment has spread to pre-hospital settings. The best-known example is defibrillators, which spread first to ambulances, then in an automatic version to police cars, and most recently to public spaces such as airports, office buildings, hotels, and even shopping malls.

Because time is such an essential factor in emergency treatment, EDs typically have their own diagnostic equipment to avoid waiting for equipment installed elsewhere in the hospital. Nearly all have an X-ray room, and many now have full radiology facilities including CT scanners and ultrasonography equipment. Laboratory services may be handled on a priority basis by the hospital lab, or the ED may have its own "STAT Lab" for basic labs (blood counts, blood typing, toxicology screens, etc.) that must be returned very rapidly.

Non-emergency Use

Metrics applicable to the ED can be grouped into three main categories, volume, cycle time, and patient satisfaction. Volume metrics including arrivals per hour, percentage of ED beds occupied and age of patients are understood at a basic level at all hospitals as an indication for staffing requirements. Cycle time metrics are the mainstays of the evaluation and tracking of process efficiency and are less widespread since an active effort is needed to collect and analyze this data.

Patient satisfaction metrics, already commonly collected by physician groups and hospitals, are useful in demonstrating the impact of changes in patient perception of care over time. Since patient satisfaction metrics are derivative and subjective, they are less useful in primary process improvement.

In many Primary Care Trusts there may be out of hours doctor services sometimes known as Keydoc or something similar (varying by area) provided by volunteer General Practitioners.

Patients attending the ED for minor complaints do not contribute significantly to the overall workload of the department. (Despite the level of complaints in the general public and by health staff.) Studies, in Australia at least, have shown that improved after-hours GP access has no effect on ED workload or waiting times.

In the United States, and many other countries, hospitals are beginning to create areas in their emergency rooms for people with minor injuries. These are commonly referred as *fast track* or Minor Care units. These units are for people with non life-threatening injuries. The use of these units within a department have been shown to significantly improve the flow of patients through a department and to reduce waiting times. Urgent care clinics are another alternative, where patients can go to receive immediate care for non-life-threatening conditions.

Doctors in Training

Doctors in training provide a large portion of the medical care in emergency departments.

In the United States, they are called residents and are supervised by ABEM board certified attending physicians.

In the United Kingdom, many doctors rotate through the emergency department, such as during their second foundation year (F2), or as part of a rotational specialty training programme in General Practice or Emergency Medicine.

Emergency Departments in the Military

Emergency departments in the military benefit from the added support of enlisted personnel who are capable of performing any task they have been trained for, regardless of actual education obtained from civilian schooling. For example, in Naval hospitals, Hospital Corpsmen perform tasks that fall under the scope of practice of both doctors (i.e. sutures and incision and drainages) and nurses (i.e. medication administration and foley catheter insertion). Often, some civilian education and/or certification will be required such as an EMT certification, in case of the need to provide care outside of the base where the member is actually stationed.

GERIATRIC INTENSIVE-CARE UNIT

Geriatric intensive care unit is a special type of intensive care unit dedicated to management of critically ill elderly.

Geriatric intensive care unit's goal is to restore physiologic stability, prevent complications, maintain comfort and safety, and preserve pre-illness functional ability and quality of life (QOL) in older adults admitted to critical-care units.

Origin

Geriatric intensive care units appeared in response to the world's population aging. Managing Geriatrics diseases is not like managing adults or pediatrics diseases, especially if they are critically ill. Geriatric medicine was not included in the curricula of undergraduate or advanced medical training until recently, so not all critical care physicians were oriented by the pecularties of geriatric patients.

Despite the fact that geriatric patients constitute many of the critically ill patients, the training of critical care team still lacks the training on the geriatrics giants.

Critically ill older adult: a person, age 65 or older, who is currently experiencing or at risk for some form of physiologic instability or alteration warranting urgent or emergent, advanced nursing/medical interventions and monitoring.

- More than half (55.8%) of all ICU days are incurred by patients older than 65.
- Older adults are living longer, are more racially and ethnically diverse, often have multiple chronic conditions, and more than one-quarter report difficulty performing one or more activities of daily living (ADLs). These factors may affect both the course and outcome of critical illness.
- Once hospitalized for a life-threatening illness, older adults often:

1. Experience high ICU, hospital, and long-term crude mortality rates.
2. Are at risk for deterioration in functional ability and post-discharge institutional care.

- Older age is also a factor that may lead to:
  1. Physician bias in refusing ICU admission.
  2. The decision to withhold mechanical ventilation, surgery, or dialysis.
  3. An increased likelihood of an established resuscitation directive.
- Most critically ill older adults:
  1. Demonstrate resiliency.
  2. Report being satisfied with their QOL post-discharge.
  3. Would reaccept ICU care and mechanical ventilation if needed.
- Chronologic age alone is not an acceptable or accurate predictor of poor outcomes after critical illness.
- Factors that may influence an older adult's ability to survive a catastrophic illness include:
  1. Severity of illness
  2. Nature and extent of co-morbidities
  3. Diagnosis, reason for/duration of mechanical ventilation
  4. Complications length of ICU/hospital stay.

Goal

Goal is to restore physiologic stability, prevent complications, maintain comfort and safety, and preserve pre-illness functional ability and quality of life (QOL) in older adults admitted to critical-care units.

Distribution in the World

Geriatric intensive care units are starting to be disseminated and are currently present in Japan, USA, China, Egypt, India & Europe (France, Italy, Poland, Germany).

Practice Issues

Critical care practice by necessity is focused on the physiological parameters of the patients being served. Thus, the most important effort revolves around maintaining physiological function and restoring homeostasis for the person who is critically ill. However, when the urgent episode subsides, inappropriate practice guidelines and clinical approaches are often used in the care of older adults.

Older individuals have less physiological reserve than younger ones and, therefore, are more likely to have dire consequences following critical care events such as cardiac or respiratory arrest. Further, there are associated geriatric syndromes, medication issues and problems that can be prevented if they are anticipated. Sleep disorders are prevalent in the elderly. During a critical care episode, sleeping and waking cycles are disturbed. Because of the noise in an ICU, less sleep and more noise may trigger delirium. Improving critical care practice for the elderly requires attention to sleep deficits, which means appropriate rest and recovery time.

Altered Eating and Feeding Patterns are commoner in geriatric intensive care units. Tubes and other devices, which can impede the ability to obtain adequate nutrition, are common in an intensive care unit. While total parenteral nutrition lines can be inserted to provide calories, the pleasure of eating is lost, as is the sensory stimulation (i.e., smell, taste, texture) of the food, which might increase appetite.

Careful attention must be paid to weight loss in the elderly during the critical care episode. Because albumin levels may already be potentially compromised, the older individual will be at risk for pressure ulcers if their nutrition falls to critically low levels. Other reasons for impaired nutrition include mouth sores; dry, cracked mouths; or a lack of dentures. These issues may be overlooked in busy units.

Foley catheters are regularly inserted in patients in the intensive care unit to monitor fluid balance, this should be changed. urinary catheters are known to cause urinary tract infections, which are potentially lethal to the elderly. Thus, when possible, catheters should be avoided in the ICU. In addition, the use of incontinence undergarments should be avoided, given the propensity for skin irritation and breakdown.

The ICU environment has been linked to delirium in the elderly. Disorientation to time or place because of overstimulation, pain and metabolic imbalances frequently results in cognitive changes. Optimally, critical care nurses must obtain a baseline mental status on the older patient upon admission and follow the changes through the use of a standardized assessment instrument such as a Mini-Mental State Examination. Early detection and intervention can reduce the use of either physical or chemical restraints.

Elderly admitted to intensive care units need special management as regard pharmacotherapy. They can suffer from special cardiovascular diseases, severe infections as MRSA of systemic fungal infections. And may need special posoperative analgesia. Also elderly need assessment by special instruments to predict the prognosis of ICU patients older than 75 years.

Ethical Issues

Geriatrics critical care dictate many ethical issues which have been put into the focus of some researches & discussions. Also visiting hours in the geriatric ICU need special organisation different from other ICUs.

Not only do critical care units utilize up to a third of hospital expenditures and about 1% of GNP, the critically ill elderly consume a disproportionate amount of ICU resources. Outcome prediction models for very elderly critically ill patients have been proposed with age as one of numerous model variables; but such models have not been widely validated. Despite the burgeoning emphasis on evidence-based population approach to health care, there is insufficient research to guide the critical care clinician. There remains a modicum of subjectivity in crucial decisions that affect the elderly patient receiving intensive care.

Older age is also one of the factors that lead to a physician bias in refusing ICU admission. Many Critical care physicians generally consider their older patients' quality of life to be worse than do the patients, although other studies that have assessed the quality of live show no age-related differences among ICU survivors. Furthermore, physicians' estimations of patient quality of life significantly influence physicians' attitudes to futility of care issues, in contrast to patients' perceptions.

Threshold for life-sustaining treatment in the elderly will continue to be different among the ICUs. Clinical decisions will be subjected to many ethical, legal, and socioeconomic pressures. Personal and religious beliefs will inevitably influence societal expectations and clinician practices. Severity of illness has the biggest influence on outcome in a critical illness. Age alone is not a predictor of short-term or long-term outcome in the older patient who is critically ill. Critical illness in the elderly remains a fertile area for future research. Also some people tend to put a stigma on the geriatric intensive-care patient in community and in games.

Some studies suggest that patients who are perceived not to benefit from critical care are more often refused intensive care unit admission;

refusal is associated with an increased risk of hospital death. During times of decreased critical bed availability, several factors, including age, illness severity, and medical diagnosis, are used to triage patients, although their relative importance is uncertain.

Some studies suggest the solution of subintensive care units. Which are now present in many places.

Training & Education Programs

Geriatric intensive care unit physicians are trained in geriatric medicine & critical care medicine. Some Universities & medical schools offer training sessions on Geritric critical care medicine. Some books focusing on older patients in the emergency department and critical care unit are available. And other online resources.

Geriatric intensive care unit nurses receive special training in critical care of elderly in their basic training, advanced and clinical training. Some Nursing school faculties are establishing research in Geriatric critical care nursing. And a Geriatric Critical Care Nursing Research (GCCNR) Group was established, the purpose of this group is to serve as a forum to share, query, and exchange ideas and strategies related to the research involving and benefiting older ICU patients.

INTENSIVE-CARE UNIT

An intensive care unit (ICU), critical care unit (CCU), intensive therapy unit or intensive treatment unit (ITU) is a specialized department used in many countries' hospitals that provides intensive care medicine. Many hospitals also have designated intensive care areas for certain specialities of medicine, as dictated by the needs and available resources of each hospital. The naming is not rigidly standardized.

History

In 1854, Florence Nightingale left for the Crimean War, where the necessity to separate seriously wounded soldiers from less-seriously wounded was observed. Nightingale reduced mortality from 40% to 2% on the battlefield, creating the concept of intensive care

In 1950, anesthesiologist Peter Safar established the concept of "Advanced Support of Life," keeping patients sedated and ventilated in an intensive care environment. Safar is considered the first intensivist.

In response to a polio epidemic (where many patients required constant ventilation and surveillance), Bjorn Ibsen established the first intensive care unit in Copenhagen in 1953. The first application of this idea in the United States was pioneered by Dr. William Mosenthal, a surgeon at the Dartmouth-Hitchcock Medical Centre. In the 1960s, the importance of cardiac arrhythmias as a source of morbidity and mortality in myocardial infarctions (heart attacks) was recognized. This led to the routine use of cardiac monitoring in ICUs, especially in the post-MI setting.

Types

Specialized types of ICUs include:

- Neonatal intensive-care unit (NICU)
- Special Care Nursery (SCN)
- Pediatric intensive-care unit (PICU)
- Psychiatric intensive-care unit (PICU)
- Coronary care unit (CCU) for heart disease
- Cardiac Surgery intensive-care unit (CSICU)
- Cardiovascular intensive-care unit (CVICU)
- Medical intensive-care unit (MICU)
- Medical Surgical intensive-care unit (MSICU)
- Surgical intensive-care unit (SICU)
- Overnight intensive recovery (OIR)
- Neuroscience/Neurotrauma intensive-care unit (NICU)
- Neurointensive-care unit (NICU)
- Burn intensive-care unit (BWICU)
- Trauma Intensive care Unit (TICU)
- Shock Trauma intensive-care unit (STICU)
- Trauma-Neuro Critical Care intensive-care unit (TNCC)
- Respiratory intensive-care unit (RICU)
- Geriatric intensive-care unit (GICU).

EQUIPMENT AND SYSTEMS

Common equipment in an ICU includes mechanical ventilator to assist breathing through an endotracheal tube or a tracheotomy opening; cardiac monitors including telemetry, external pacemakers, and defibrillators; dialysis equipment for renal problems; equipment for the constant monitoring of bodily functions; a web of intravenous lines, feeding tubes, nasogastric tubes, suction pumps, drains and catheters; and a wide array of drugs to treat the main condition(s). Medically induced comas, analgesics, and induced sedation reduce pain and prevent secondary infections.

Quality of Care

Medicine suggests a relation between ICU volume and quality of care for mechanically ventilated patients. After adjustment for severity of illness, demographic variables, and characteristics of the ICUs (including staffing by intensivists), higher ICU volume was significantly associated with lower ICU and hospital mortality rates. Typically, patient to nurse ratio is what determines the care. A ratio of 2 patients to 1 nurse is recommended for a medical ICU. This is unlike the ratio of 4:1 or 5:1 ratio on the medical floors.

Staff

Medical staff typically includes intensivists with training in internal medicine, surgery, anesthesia, or emergency medicine. Many nurse practitioners and physician assistants with specialized training are also now part of the staff that provide continuity of care for patients. Staff typically includes specially trained critical care registered nurses, registered respiratory therapists, clinical pharmacists, nutritionists, physical therapists, certified nursing assistants, social workers etc.

Intensive Care Around the World

In the United Kingdom intensive care medicine is an extremely specialised area. In the United States up to 20% of hospital beds can be labelled as intensive care beds, whereas in the United Kingdom intensive care usually will comprise only up to 2% of total beds. This high disparity is attributed to patients in the UK who are admitted to an ICU tending to be only the most severely ill.

Intensive Care is an incredibly expensive healthcare service. In the United Kingdom the average cost of funding an intensive care unit is:

- £838 per bed per day for a Neonatal Intensive Care Unit
- £1,702 per bed per day for a Pediatric Intensive Care Unit
- £1,328 per bed per day for an Adult Intensive Care Unit

ICU QUALITY AND MANAGEMENT TOOLS

The intensive care unit (ICU) is one of the major components of the current health care system. The advances in supportive care and monitoring resulted in significant improvements in the care of surgical and clinical patients. Nowadays aggressive surgical therapies as well as transplantation are made safer by the monitoring in a closed environment, the surgical ICU, in the post-operative period. Moreover, the care and full recovery of many severely ill clinical patients as those with life-threatening infections occurs as a result of intensive care.

However, despite many significant advances in various fields as mechanical ventilation, renal replacement therapy, antimicrobial therapy and hemodynamic monitoring this increased knowledge and the wise use of such technology is not available for all patients. Shortage of ICU beds are an important issue, however even when ICU beds are available significant variability in treatment and in the adherence to evidence-based interventions do not occur.

Tools for ICU Quality Monitoring

Several measures of ICU performance have been proposed in the past 30 years. It is intuitive, and correct, to assume that ICU mortality may be a useful marker of quality. However, crude mortality rates does not take into consideration the singular aspects of each specific patient population that is treated in a certain geographic region, hospital or ICU. Therefore approaches looking for standardized mortality ratios that are adjusted for disease severity, comorbidities and other clinical aspects are often sought. Severity of illness is usually evaluated by scoring systems that integrates clinical, physiologic and demographic variables. Scoring systems are interesting tools to describe ICU populations and explain their different outcomes. The most frequently used are the APACHE II, SAPS II and MPM. However, newer scores as APACHE IV and SAPS III have been recently introduced in clinical practice. More than only using scoring systems, one should search for a high rate of adherence to clinically effective interventions. Adherence to interventions as deep venous thrombosis prophylaxis, reduction of ICU-acquired infections, adequate sedation regimens and decreasing and reporting serious adverse events are essential and have been accepted as benchmarking of quality.

The complex task of collecting and analyzing data on performance measures are made easier when clinical information systems are available. Although several clinical information systems focus on important aspects as computerized physician order entry systems and individual patient tracking information, few have attempted to gather clinical information generating full reports that provide a panorama of the ICU performance and detailed data on several domains as mortality, length of stay, severity of illness, clinical scores, nosocomial infections, adverse events and adherence to good clinical practice. Through implementing quality initiatives, increasing the quality of care and patient safety are major and feasible goals. Such systems (for example: Epimed Monitor) are available for clinical use and may facilitate the process of care on a daily basis and provide data for an in-depth analysis of ICU performance.

Neonatal Intensive-care Unit

A neonatal intensive care unit, usually shortened NICU (sometimes pronounced "Nickyou") and also called a newborn intensive care unit, intensive care nursery (ICN), and special care baby unit (SCBU [pronounced "Skiboo"], especially in Great Britain), or a humidicrib, is a unit of a hospital specializing in the care of ill or premature newborn infants. The NICU is distinct from a special care nursery (SCN) in providing a high level of intensive care to premature infants while the SCN provides specialized care for infants with less severe medical problems.

NICUs were developed in the 1950s and 1960s by pediatricians to provide better temperature support, isolation from infection risk, specialized feeding, and greater access to specialized equipment and resources. Infants are cared for in incubators or "open warmers."

Some low birth weight infants need respiratory support ranging from extra oxygen (by head hood or nasal cannula) to continuous positive airway pressure (CPAP) or mechanical ventilation. Public access is limited, and staff and visitors are required to take precautions to reduce transmission of infection. Nearly all children's hospitals have NICUs, but they can often be found in large general hospitals as well. A NICU is typically directed by one or more neonatologists and staffed by nurses, nurse practitioners, Nursery Nurses, physician assistants, resident physicians, and respiratory therapists. Many other ancillary services are necessary for a top-level NICU. Other physicians, especially those with "organ-defined" specialties often assist in the care of these infants.

EQUIPMENT

Incubator

An *incubator* (or *open warmer* or *isolette*) is an apparatus used to maintain environmental conditions suitable for a neonate, (newborn baby). It is used in preterm births.

Possible functions of a neonatal incubator are:

- Oxygenation, through oxygen supplementation by head hood or nasal cannula, or even continuous positive airway pressure (CPAP) or mechanical ventilation. Infant respiratory distress syndrome is the leading cause of death in preterm infants, and the main treatments are CPAP, in addition to administering surfactant and stabilizing the blood sugar, blood salts, and blood pressure.
- Observation: Modern neonatal intensive care involves sophisticated measurement of temperature, respiration, cardiac function, oxygenation, and brain activity.
- Protection from cold temperature, infection, noise, drafts and excess handling: Incubators may be described as bassinets enclosed in plastic, with climate control equipment designed to keep them warm and limit their exposure to germs.
- Provision of nutrition, through intravenous catheters
- Administration of medications.
- Maintaining fluid balance by providing fluid and keeping a high air humidity to prevent a too great loss from skin and respiratory evaporation.

A *transport incubator* is an incubator and the most necessary neonatal instruments in a transportable format, and is used when a sick or premature baby is moved, e.g. from one hospital to another, as from a community hospital to a larger medical centre with a proper neonatal intensive care unit.

It usually has a miniature ventilator, cardio-respiratory monitor, IV pump, pulse oximeter, and oxygen supply built into its frame.

Early years

Doctors took an increasing role in childbirth from the eighteenth century onwards. However, the care of newborn babies, sick or well, remained largely in the hands of mothers and midwives. Some baby incubators, similar to those used for hatching chicks, were devised in the late nineteenth century. In the United States these were shown at commercial exhibitions, complete with babies inside, until 1943. It wasn't until after the Second World War that special care baby units (SCBUs) were established in many hospitals. In Britain, early SCBUs opened in Birmingham and Bristol. At Southmead Hospital, Bristol, initial opposition from obstetricians lessened after quadruplets born there in 1948 were successfully cared for in the new unit. More resources became available - the first unit had been set up with £100. Most early units had little equipment and relied on careful nursing and observation.

Incubators were expensive so the whole room often was kept warm instead. Cross-infection between babies was greatly feared. Strict nursing routines involved staff wearing gowns and masks, constant hand washing and minimal handling of babies. Parents were sometimes allowed to watch through the windows of the unit. Much was learned about feeding - frequent, tiny feeds seemed best - and breathing. Oxygen was given freely until the end of the 1950s, when it was shown that the high concentrations reached inside incubators caused some babies to go blind. Monitoring conditions in the incubator, and the baby itself, was to become a major area of research. Although incubators provided oxygen and warmth, science in the 1950s was limited and it was not until later that technology played a larger role in the decline of infant mortality. Even though the elimination of infectious disease was mostly responsible for decline in infant mortality, low birth weight infant mortality remained high. Yet, because of medical advances in neonatology, low birth weight infants today are surviving on average 15 years more than low weight infants born in the 1950s.

Increasing Technology

By the 1970s SCBUs were an established part of hospitals in the developed world. In Britain, some early units ran community programmes, sending experienced nurses to help care for premature babies at home. But increasingly technological monitoring and therapy meant special care for babies became hospital-based. By the 1980s, over 90% of births took place in hospital anyway. The emergency dash from home to SCBU with baby in a transport incubator had become a thing of the past, though transport incubators were still needed. Specialist equipment and expertise were not available at every hospital, and strong arguments were made for large, centralised SCBUs. On the downside was the long travelling time for frail babies and for parents. A 1979 study showed that 20% of babies in SCBUs for up to a week were never visited by either parent. Centralised or not, by the 1980s few questioned the role of SCBUs in saving babies. Around 80% of babies born weighing under 1.5 kg now survived, compared to around 40% in the 1960s. From 1982 in Britain pediatricians could train and qualify in the sub-specialty of neonatal medicine.

Not only careful nursing, but also new techniques and instruments now played a major role. As in adult intensive care units, the use of monitoring and life support systems became routine. These needed special modification for small babies, whose bodies were tiny and often immature. Adult ventilators, for example, could damage babies lungs and gentler techniques with smaller pressure changes were devised. The many tubes and sensors used for monitoring the baby's condition, blood sampling and artificial feeding made some babies scarcely visible beneath the technology.

Furthermore, by 1975, over 18% of newborn babies in Britain were being admitted to SCBUs. Some hospitals admitted all babies delivered by Caesarian section, or under 2500g in weight. The fact that these babies missed early close contact with their mothers was a growing concern. As in other area of medicine, the 1980s saw questions being raised about the human, and the economic costs of too much technology. Admission policies gradually changed. In addition, treating low birth weight infants is expensive, especially when there are much cheaper ways of ensuring healthy babies. The key is prevention. Money can be spent on programs educating mothers on staying healthy during their pregnancy. One program (one that encourages women to stop smoking) is one third the price of neonatal intensive care and has been proven to work. During this program, a significant number of women often quit.

Changing Priorities

SCBUs now concentrate on treating very small, premature, or otherwise sick babies. Some of these babies are from higher-order multiple births, but most are still single babies born too early. Premature labour, and how to prevent it, remains a perplexing problem for doctors. Even though medical advancements allow doctors to save low birth weight babies, it is almost invariably better to delay such births.

Over the last 10 years or so, SCBUs have become much more 'parent friendly', encouraging maximum involvement with the babies. Routine gowns and masks have gone and parents are encouraged to help with care as much as possible. Cuddling, and skin-to-skin contact, also known as Kangaroo care, are seen as beneficial for all but the frailest (very tiny babies are exhausted by the stimulus of being handled, or larger critically ill infants). Less stressful ways of delivering high-technology medicine to tiny patients have been devised - stick-on sensors to measure blood oxygen levels through the skin, for example, and ways of reducing the amount of blood taken for tests.

Some major problems of the SCBU have almost disappeared. Exchange transfusions, in which all the blood is removed and replaced, little by little, are rare now. Rhesus incompatibility (a difference in blood groups) between mother and baby is largely preventable. Breathing difficulties and brain hemorrhage still claim many infant lives and are the focus of many current research projects.

The long term outlook for premature babies saved by SCBUs has always been a concern. From the early years, it was reported that a higher proportion than normal grew up with disabilities, including cerebral palsy and learning difficulties. Now that treatments are available for many of the problems faced by tiny or immature babies in the first weeks of life, long-term follow-up, and minimising long-term disability, are major research areas.

Besides prematurity and extreme low birth weight, common diseases cared for in a NICU include perinatal asphyxia, extreme cases of preeclampsia/eclampsia, major birth defects, sepsis, neonatal jaundice, and respiratory distress syndrome due to immaturity of the lungs. The leading cause of death in NICUs is generally necrotizing enterocolitis. Complications of extreme prematurity may include intracranial hemorrhage, chronic bronchopulmonary dysplasia, or retinopathy of prematurity. An infant may spend a day of observation in a NICU or may spend many months there. Overall survival rates, for all gestational ages lumped together, are roughly 70%.

Neonatology and NICUs have greatly increased the survival of very low birth weight and extremely premature infants. In the era before NICUs, infants of birth weight less than 1400 grams (3 lb, usually about 30 weeks gestation) rarely survived. Today, infants of 500 grams at 26 weeks have a fair chance of survival.

The NICU environment provides challenges as well as benefits. Stressors for the infants can include continual light, a high level of noise, separation from their mothers, reduced physical contact, painful procedures, and interference with the opportunity to breastfeed. A NICU can be stressful for the staff as well. A special aspect of NICU stress for both parents and staff is that infants may survive, but with damage to the brain or eyes.

NICU rotations are essential aspects of pediatric and obstetric residency programs, but NICU experience is encouraged by other specialty residencies, such as family practice, surgery, Pharmacy, and emergency medicine.

7

Application of Standards for Health Promotion in Hospitals

Application of existing standard and criteria in hospitals has not led to noticeable results. Also, the integration and productivity of existing standard does not facilitate health development and promotion. Therefore, designing the standards for health promotion activities in hospitals is required. Putting stronger emphasis on working conditions in hospitals is needed so as to improve the health of staff, and efficiency and quality of care. Setting standards is the main strategy to improve quality in health care. However, a review of the main standards in use by accreditation agencies yielded few standards related to health promotion actions.

Recognizing the need for standards for health promotion in hospitals, WHO established a working group at the ninth International Conference on health promoting hospitals, Copenhagen, May 2001. Thereafter, several working groups and country networks have been working on the development of standards. After these three workshops, the standards for health promotion in hospitals are considered to be in their final format (subject to future revision once new evidence emerges). It can be said that due to the nature of these standards that today's role and responsibility of hospitals is health promotion of patient, staff, organization and community.

Finally, five standards were developed addressing the following issues:

Standard 1: Management policy: Demand that a hospital has a written policy for health promotion. This policy must be implemented as part of the overall organization quality system and is aiming to improve health outcome. It is stated that the policy is aimed at patient, relatives and staff.

Standard 2: Patient assessment: Describes the organizations' obligation to ensure the assessment of the patients' needs for health promotion, disease prevention and rehabilitation.

Standard 3: Patient information and intervention: States that the organization must provide the patient with information on significant factors concerning their disease or health condition and health promotion interventions should be established in all patients' pathways.

Standard 4: Promoting a healthy workplace: It gives the management the responsibility to establish conditions for the development of the hospital as a healthy workplace.

Standard 5: Continuity and cooperation: Demanding a planned approach to collaboration with other health service sectors and institutions.

Materials And Methods

This study was a descriptive - analytical survey in selected hospitals of Iran (38 hospitals from 4 provinces: Tehran, Esfahan, shiraz, Gilan). Method of data collecting was through reviewing documentation related to each of the standards. WHOs self-assessment tool for health promotion was used for data collection. Each standard has substandards. Substandards operationalize the standard and break it down into its principle components. There are overall 24 substandards; the number of substandards per standards varies from 4 to 6. Content validity was considered for instrument validity. Reliability was calculated via Cronbach's alpha (r = 0.78).

Evidence for evaluation

To collect data documentation related to each of the standard some documents were reviewed. A sample of reviewed documents for each of standards is explained below;

Standard 1: Management policy: Strategic planning for mentioned health promotion concepts in the mission and vision statement, agreement with other organizations such as the Ministry of Health to participate in the HPH project, The hospital's quality and business plans including HPH concept, existing guidelines for action related to patients, specific plan for staff and community, staff member nominated for the coordination of HPH plans, reviewing annual performance evaluation or staff's participation in the HP program, reviewing newsletters, posters or brochures related HP, training program on HP.

Standard 2: Patient assessment: Availability of patient health promotion needs assessment guidelines, review of patient records. The date of patient assessment which is written down in the patient record, and availability of Information from referring physician or other relevant sources in the patients record.

Standard 3: Patient information and intervention: Random review of patient records for all patients, availability of general health and high-risk disease information, doing various assessment methods: survey, focused group with managers, interview with staff, questionnaire.

Standard 4: Healthy workplace: Interviews with new staff for HP training, Availability of smoking cessation programs, Availability of policy for healthy food, checking food offered in canteen, checking questionnaire used for staff's knowledge on health promotion, checking minutes of working groups for participation of staff representatives. Availability of staffs annual assessment program about HP, checking with staff for participating in the seminar.

Standard 5: Continuity and cooperation: Interviewing with management board making sure of their awareness toward the health plan, availability of review documents related to health programs and documenting their references, patients' evaluation assessed in patient surveys, existence of specific rehabilitation programs for patients, list of health organizations colleague in the hospital, existence of programs and activities after patient discharge. Availability of procedures for the exchange of information with other health care organizations that take account of patient confidentiality, reviewing patient's medical records for rehabilitation programs.

Data analysis

Data analysis was performed through statistical indicators (mean, SD) and *t*-test, paired *t*-test. Sample of research was government and private hospitals in 5 provinces in Iran.

Results

Overall the mean score of health promotion standard in the state hospital was 54.1 ± 15.1 showing that the private hospitals have higher score. In general, patient Information and intervention standard had the highest score (70.8 ± 8.1), both in private and government hospitals. Score of this standard in private hospitals was (75 ± 8.6) and in government hospitals was (69 ± 9.4). Based on these results the private hospitals have been better. In this standard, substandards 3-1 and 3-4 had the highest standard and the patient assessment standard had the lowest score (44.2 ± 20.1). Score of this standard in private hospitals was (43.5 ± 5.1) and in government hospitals was (44.4 ± 24. 6). Clearly also in this standard, private hospitals have been better in this standard, substandards 2-3 and 2-4 had the lowest standard. Continuity and cooperation standard had the lowest score among the government hospitals, which in this standard, substandards 5-2 and 5-4 had the lowest standard. Patient assessment standard had the lowest score among the private hospitals, which in this standard, and the need assessment for health promotion for diagnosis-related patient-groups substandard had the lowest standard. T-test showed that there is no significant difference of mean score of S1 until S4 among government and private hospitals. However, significantly the S5 mean score in private hospitals were higher than government hospitals.

Repeated measure of ANOVA showed that the mean scores of different standards of health promoting were not equal in hospitals (F = 16.4, *P* = 0.00).

As seen in Table 3 highest scores are related to the S3, S1 and S4 are located in the second grade and S2 and S5 have been in the third grade. Also, T-paired test showed that S1 and S4 standards are not significantly different together also no significant difference between S2 and S5, but significantly S3 mean score is more than the rest standard. And also significantly S1 and S4 have higher score than S2 and S5 .

Discussion

Overall the mean score of health promotion standard in the hospitals was 54.1 ± 15.1, showing that the private hospitals had higher score. And in general the patient information and intervention standard had the highest score (70.8 ± 8.1). This suggests that the hospitals have a strong information system of patients and their family and patients are given clear, understandable and appropriate information about their condition, treatment, care and factors influencing their health. This standard both in private and government hospitals had the highest score, and the patient assessment standard had lower score (44.2 ± 20.1). This suggests a lack of clear systems and procedures regarding the determination and evaluation of patient's health promotion needed in hospitals. may be a hospital has a program for patient assessment but in this assessment does not pay attention to social and cultural issues governmental hospitals had a lower score in continuity and cooperation standard.

This shows that governmental hospitals do not identify and cooperate with existing health and social care providers, related organizations and groups in the community and do not implement activities and procedures after patient discharge as *t*-test showed that significantly the mean score of S5 in private hospitals were higher than government hospitals.

In fact, private hospitals had a clear plan in providing services after discharge, time, procedures of cooperation with other organizations and information exchange procedures. Also, they documented the interventions. One important element in creating a health promoting hospital is training to staff and patients in improving and implementing health promotion. This issue is one of the elements of S1 (Management Policy) in health promotion standards and is emphasized in many studies. Researchers have expressed four domains for health promotion in the hospital (patient - oriented, staff-oriented, organization and community- oriented). In this study a WHO health promoting hospital tool was used which is also emphasized on above domain. So it is similar to another research.

Johnson offers four different types of organizational approaches to HPH. In the best type, the hospital is improving health promotion of patient, staff, organization and community. Also WHO concerned that a HPH is improving health promotion of patient, staff, organization and community. The issue has observed in the questionnaire that was used. Research shows that hospitals that get accreditation certificate, have a planning for improving health promotion for patient, staff, organization and community. In fact, these hospitals have comprehensive services, also the check list used in this research considers health promotion for patient, staff, organization and community. To use WHO -HPH tools in the other countries of Africa or Asia this research is needed to be redesigned. This tool was edited considering the culture of patients and the health system in Iran.

Richardson expressed that the hospital environments would not seem as centers of excellence'. Also this research in a s4 (promoting a healthy workplace) has emphasized this issue. One of the main obstacles against the development of HPH is shortage of supplies, personnel, training, time, managers understanding of the concept and principles of health promotion in hospital and professional skills. This paper has considered above cases in evaluation hospitals as a HPH. Peter Olden has stated management as one of the stages of health promotion implementation. This issue is expressed in a S1 (management policy) that was used in this paper. Two strategies for improving health promotion are education and experimental classes Education as one important element in this study is standard 1 (management policy).

HEALTH PROMOTION: DEFINITION AND CONCEPT

Health promotion measures focus on both individuals and on contextual factors that shape the actions of individuals with the aim to prevent and reduce ill health and improve wellbeing. Health in this context not only refers to the traditional, objective and biomedical view of the absence of infirmity or disease but to a holistic view that adds mental resources and social well-being to physical health. Health promotion goes beyond health education and disease prevention, in as far as it is based on the concept of salutogenesis and stresses the analysis and development of the health potential of individuals.

The scope of *disease prevention* has been defined in the Health Promotion Glossary as "measures not only to prevent the occurrence of disease, such as risk factor reduction, but also to arrest its progress and reduce its consequences once established". The same source defines the scope of *health education* as comprising "consciously constructed opportunities for learning involving some form of communication designed to improve health literacy, including improving knowledge and developing life skills which are conducive to individual and community health". Health promotion is defined as a broader concept in the WHO Ottawa Charter as "the process of enabling people to increase control over, and improve, their health".

In practice, these terms are frequently used complementarily and measures for the implementation may overlap; however, there are major conceptual differences with regard to the focus and impact of health promotion actions.

Whereas the medical approach is directed at physiological risk factors (e.g. high blood pressure, immunization status), the behavioural approach is directed at lifestyle factors (e.g. smoking, physical inactivity) and the socio-environmental approach is directed at general conditions (such as unemployment, low education or poverty). Health promotion consequently includes, but goes far beyond medical approaches directed at curing individuals.

Based on the notion of health as a positive concept, the Ottawa Charter put forward the idea that "health is created and lived by people within the settings of their everyday life; where they learn, work, play and love". This settings approach to health promotion, founded on the experience of community and organizational development, led to a number of initiatives such as Health Promoting Cities, Health Promoting Schools, and Health Promoting Hospitals, etc. in order to improve people's health where they spend most of their time: in organizations.

The settings approach acknowledges that behavioural changes are only possible and stable if they are integrated into everyday life and correspond with concurrent habits and existing cultures.

Health Promotion interventions in organizations therefore not only have to address changing individuals but also underlying norms, rules and cultures. The Ottawa Charter identifies five priority action areas for health promotion:

- Build healthy public policy: health promotion policy combines diverse but complementary approaches, including legislation, fiscal measures, taxation and organization change. Health promotion policy requires the identification of obstacles to the adoption of healthy public policies in non-health sectors and the development of ways to remove them.
- Create supportive environments for health: the protection of the natural and build environments and the conservation of natural resources must be addressed in any health promotion strategy.
- Strengthen community action for health: Community development draws on existing human and material resources to enhance self-help and social support, and to develop flexible systems for strengthening public participation in, and direction of, health matters. This requires full and continuous access to information and learning opportunities for health, as well as funding support.
- Develop personal skills: Enabling people to learn (throughout life) to prepare themselves for all stages and to cope with chronic illness and injuries is essential. This has to be facilitated in school, home, work and community settings.
- Re-orient health services: the role of the health sector must move increasingly in a health promotion direction, beyond its responsibility for providing clinical and curative services. Reorientation of health services also requires stronger attention to health research, as well as changes in professional education and training.

The Impact of Health Services on Health

Many health professionals presume that health promotion has always been the core business of medicine in general and hospitals in particular. This view may be challenged for a variety of reasons. Although the history goes back further, the first identifiable hospitals were built during the 12th century and were religious-oriented, cloister-affiliated institutions providing support to the poor, elderly, psychologically deviant and others in need. In the foreground were the accommodation, nourishment and the isolation of infectious diseases, not the treatment of disease.

Until the late 19th century hospitals were not a place where health was created, but rather a place to die. This changed with the development of the science of medicine, supported by utilitarian state philosophy and humanism. Since then, the potential of hospital care to improve health has made rapid improvements with the development of aseptic and antiseptic techniques, more effective anaesthesia, greater surgical knowledge and skills, trauma techniques, blood transfusion, coronary artery bypass surgery, effective pharmaceuticals, transplantation techniques and minimal invasive surgery.

However, parallel to the advances in hospital procedures, questions have been raised with regard to the contribution of health care to the health of the population and the effectiveness of health care services. Various accounts have been made discarding the claims of health care for the reduction of infectious diseases, the significant decline in infant mortality, reductions in the major causes of death and resulting increase in life expectancy.

Although controversy is still continuing on details of his work, McKeown demonstrated compellingly how reductions in mortality in the United Kingdom, which were thought to be related to accomplishments of medical care, were in fact related to improvements in hygiene and nutrition. Another perspective was brought in by Ivan Illich and Rick Carlson who argued that medical care is more a cause of death, than of health. According to Illich, medicine has the potential to cause as much harm as good, as reflected in his concept of *iatrogenesis*. He strongly criticized the medical professions of their "sick-making powers" and contended that health care institutions performed the opposite of their original purpose. Carlson argued along the same lines and forecasted that the limited effectiveness of medicine will further decline in the future. Recently, these perspectives gained a lot of prominence with the report of the Institute of Medicine, "To err is human", which estimates that in the USA about 100,000 deaths in hospitals annually are due to medical errors.

A more operational perspective was brought in by the Avedis Donabedian and others who, being well aware of the limited population impact of health care, focused on strategies to improve the quality of health care services. Although major advances have been made with the outcomes movement and health technology assessment, the definition of quality as doing the right thing and doing it well, still raises fundamental questions and points to potential improvements in the provision of health care services.

The Health Promoting Hospitals network links the various perspectives above. It is driven by the strong perception that hospital services need to be more targeted towards the need of people, and not only to their organs or physiological parameters, in order to have a more substantial and lasting impact on health. At the same time the HPH philosophy is now based on strong evidence and methods to incorporate health promotion as a core principle in the organization. Quality strategies already applied in clinical settings and for the management of health care organizations are applicable to health promotion as well. Before addressing this issue further below, the following paragraphs provide the rationale for and concrete examples of health promotion services in hospitals.

Health Promotion Activities in Hospitals

Given the scope of possible health promotion interventions in hospitals, the WHO HPH movement focuses on four areas: promoting the health of patients, promoting the health of staff, changing the organization to a health promoting setting, and promoting the health of the community in the catchment area of the hospital. These four areas are reflected in the definition of a health promoting hospital:

"A *health promoting hospital* does not only provide high quality comprehensive medical and nursing services, but also develops a corporate identity that embraces the aims of health promotion, develops a health promoting organizational structure and culture, including active, participatory roles for patients and all members of staff, develops itself into a health promoting physical environment, and actively cooperates with its community".

There is a large scope and public health impact for offering health promotion strategies in health care settings. Hospitals consume between

40% and 70% of the national health care expenditure and typically employ about 1% to 3% of the working population. These working places, most of which are occupied by women, are characterized by certain physical, chemical, biological and psychosocial risk factors. Paradoxically, in hospitals – organizations that aim to restore health – the acknowledgement of factors that endanger the health of their staff is poorly developed. Health promotion programmes can improve the health of staff, reduce absenteeism rates, and improve productivity and quality.

Health professionals in hospitals can also have a lasting impact on influencing the behaviour of patients and relatives, who are more responsive to health advice in situations of experienced ill-health. This is of particular importance for two reasons: firstly, the prevalence of chronic diseases (e.g. diabetes, cardiovascular diseases, cancer) is increasing in Europe and throughout the world; secondly, many hospital treatments today not only prevent premature death but improve the quality of life of patients. In order to maintain this quality, the patient's own behaviour after discharge and effective support from relatives are important variables. Health Promotion Programmes can encourage healthy behaviour, prevent readmission and maintain quality of life of patients.

Hospitals also typically produce high amounts of waste and hazardous substances. Introducing Health Promotion strategies in hospitals can help reduce the pollution of the environment and the cooperation with other institutions and professionals can help achieve the highest possible coordination of care. Furthermore, as research and teaching institutions hospital produce, accumulate and disseminate a lot of knowledge and they can have an impact on the local health structures and influence professional practice elsewhere.

EVIDENCE FOR GENERAL HEALTH PROMOTION

There is documentation for the effect of health promotion in relation to lifestyle factors.

Tobacco

Tobacco causes a wide range of diseases. Smoking causes 30% of all occurrences of ischaemic heart disease, explains 90% of lung cancer, 75% of chronic obstructive lung disease (smoker's lungs) and 6 % of hip fracture. Not only do diseases occur more frequently in smokers, they also occur at a younger age compared to non-smokers. And population studies show that there are twice as many admissions among smokers as among non-smokers. A great number of hospital admissions are related to patients' lifestyles. Tobacco related diseases cause 30% of all admissions in an ordinary medical ward. And in addition, tobacco plays an indirect role for many other admissions. Smoking also influences the outcome of treatment. It is well documented that medical treatment for hypertension, radiation treatment of cancers of the head and the neck, treatment of arteriosclerosis and wounds are much less effective in smokers than in non-smokers. Smoking influences the immune system and plays a role in the prolongation of hospital stay for patients with infections.

Patients' long term condition and prognosis are also influenced. There is documentation that patients who stop smoking following myocardial infarction diminish the risk of recurrence within the following two years by 50%.

Unplanned readmissions cause considerable expenditure for the health care sector. Smokers have almost twice as many readmissions as non-smokers. Studies show that the average rate of readmission amounts to between 16% and 27%; patients with ischaemic heart disease, smokers' lungs (COPD) and lung cancer have a particular high rate of readmissions.

Smoking cessation has a well-documented effect on symptoms and health. Many studies show a dose-response relation between exposure to tobacco (duration of smoking habit and amount smoked) and the occurrence of disease. Similarly, there is direct proportional relationship between how long a person has been smoke free and a reduced risk of disease. Recent studies document that even smoking cessation at the age of 65 has a positive effect on health and reduces morbidity, however, a reduction of the amount consumed plays no decisive role.

In short, documentation shows that smoking cessation:

- reduces or removes lung diseases such as coughing and expectorate in healthy smokers;
- normalizes future loss of lung function in patients with established chronic lung disease;
- reduces by half the risk of cancers after 5 years (former large scale smokers do, however, have an increased risk of lung cancer for the rest of their lives);
- leads to an immediate drop in the risk of cardiac and cerebral infarction;
- reduces by half the risk of another infarction and of death within the years following acute myocardial infarction;

- reduces the risk of arteriosclerosis and related diseases;
- reduces the risk of osteoporosis and resulting hip fracture;
- reduces the risk of giving birth to a premature infant if undertaken during the first 3 to 4 months of pregnancy;
- reduces the risk of late complications in patients with diabetes;
- improves the delayed healing process of wound and tissue healing.

The evidence is based upon descriptive studies of smoking and randomized clinical studies of stop smoking, giving a high level of evidence.

Alcohol

Large scale alcohol consumption adds to the risk of diseases such as pneumonia, infections, diarrhoea and malabsorption, dissemination of cancer, non-alcoholic liver disease, hypertension, poorly regulated diabetes, fluid and electrolyte imbalances. Patients with a high alcohol intake are more often admitted to hospital; about 20% of men and 10% of the women admitted to hospital consume alcohol in excess of internationally recommended limits. Patients' alcohol consumption also influences the outcome of treatment and care. The mechanisms include reduced immune function, sub clinical or clinical cardiac dysfunction, haemostatic imbalance, delayed healing of wound and slow tissue and bone turnover, myopathy, and increased stress-response; all contribute to prolongation of hospital stay for the patients. There is evidence that cessation and to some degree reduction of alcohol consumption leads to:

- fewer admissions with alcohol related disorders such as cirrhosis of the liver and Pancreatitis;
- fewer admissions due to poisoning, alcoholism and alcohol psychosis;
- fewer infections (especially pneumonia and tuberculosis);
- improved wound and bone healing;
- improved heart function and blood pressure;
- improved outcome for several non-alcoholic diseases (among other effects).

The evidence is based upon descriptive studies of alcohol intake and randomized clinical studies of stop drinking as well as randomized studies of voluntary excessive alcohol intake, giving a high level of evidence.

Physical Activity

Lack of physical activity is associated with increased occurrence of type 2 diabetes, overweight, high blood fat levels, hypertension and development of metabolic syndrome. There is evidence that regular physical activity:

- reduces the risk of developing cardiovascular disease in general and ischaemic heart disease in particular;
- reduces the risk of developing type 2 diabetes;
- reduces mortality in middle-aged and elderly persons of both sexes;
- strengthens the development of bone density, restrains age related drop in bone mineral content and prevents the development of osteoporosis;
- prevents hypertension and reduces hypertension;
- prevents overweight;
- prevents depression, reduces tension and increases self-respect;
- prevents loss of muscle mass in elderly patients and reduces the risk of falls.

Physical training is an important element in several rehabilitation programmes, e.g. cardiac rehabilitation, rehabilitation of chronic obstructive lung disease, surgical rehabilitation, psychiatric rehabilitation etc.

Physical training for patients with myocardial infarction reduces the risk of another infarction by 25% in the first three years. Training is also an important element in mobilization of patients with rheumatoid arthritis and patients with arthritis, and studies have shown that exercise in the form of walks may put off the time of surgical intervention for patients who are waiting for knee or hip replacement. The evidence is based upon descriptive studies of physical activity and randomized clinical studies, giving a high level of evidence.

Nutrition

In the European population, overweight is the most common health problem. The increasing prevalence of overweight leads to a growing number of persons with diabetes, cardiovascular disease, strain injury and hormone related cancers. However, a problem encountered by hospitals is under-nourishment. Studies show that almost 30 % of hospital patients are undernourished on admission. At the same time, studies show that patients' food intake during hospital stay often amounts to only 60% of their actual needs. There is documentation that undernourished patients have increased morbidity and mortality than well-nourished patients. At the same time, there is documentation that systematic screening of nutrition status and proper nutritional therapy during admission reduce the risk of wound infection and lead to shorter hospital stay and contribute to more rapid convalescence. There is evidence that nutritional interventions in relation to undernourished patients:

- improve lung functions and walking distance in patients with chronic lung disease;
- increase weight and muscle mass in patients with cancer;
- increase physical activity and reduces mortality in geriatric patients;
- reduce mortality in patients with acute renal failure.

The evidence is based upon several randomized clinical studies, giving a high level of evidence.

Recommendations with Regard to Hospital Tasks

There is international consensus that patients should be given recommendations, guidance and support with regard to health promotion in hospitals. Health promotion secures that risk conditions are identified and that the patient has knowledge of the significance of these conditions, recommendations for changes and active support for carrying out these changes. Evidence exists for the following interventions, which should be implemented in general hospital practice:

Tobacco

- identification of smokers and establishing a thorough tobacco history;
- oral and written information to patients on damaging effects and health benefits, and the possibility of smoking cessation;
- advice and recommendations with regard to cessation;
- establishing smoking cessation services or integration of smoking cessation counselling as part of treatment.

Alcohol

- identification of patients with harmful and dependent alcohol consumption according to ICD-10 criteria;
- oral and written information to patients on damaging effects and health benefits and the possibilities of assistance to stop or reducing consumption;
- recommendations for large scale consumers to stop or reduce consumption;

- offering brief interventions (for harmful intake) or referral to alcohol unit (for dependent intake).

Physical Activity

- identification of patients with a need for counselling on physical activity;
- counselling on exercise in accordance with international guidelines, and followup and counselling in connection with subsequent contacts with the department;
- establishing systematic training programmes for relevant patients (heart and lung patients, diabetes, surgery, psychiatry, overweight and underweight).

Nutrition

- identification of undernourished patients and patients at risk of undernourishment;
- initiation of relevant nutrition treatment and continued observation of body weight and food intake throughout the patient's stay in hospital;
- communication of information on discharge (to own doctor, home care, general practitioner);
- identification of overweight patients and screening for diabetes and other complications;
- counselling on diet and physical training;
- establishing of systematic training programmes for relevant patients;
- secure follow up in the primary health care sector.

SYSTEMATIC INTERVENTION AND PATIENT EDUCATION

The aim of health counselling is to support the individual's process of change with regard to lifestyle. Health counselling is based on theories of behavioural change.

The theories describe the phases and processes that people go through when they change behaviour. The model describes behavioural change as a circular process. Most people go through the process several times before they finally change behaviour. Health counselling consists of a dialogue with the patient and is based on:

- the patient's knowledge of the influence of tobacco and alcohol on health and the significance of cessation/reduction for disease, treatment and health;
- the patient's ideas, emotions and attitudes with regard to the consumption under consideration;
- the patient's previous experiences when trying to change habits;
- recognition of the patient's emotions with regard to consumption;
- acceptance of the patient's choice with regard to consumption and;
- setting realistic goals for the outcome of the interview that correspond to the phase of change that the patient is going through.

There is evidence that health counselling may be used to motivate lifestyle changes. Since 1996, the Bispebjerg Hospital (Copenhagen, Denmark) has been trying to develop systematic intervention with regard to alcohol and tobacco, which includes health counselling for all patients including outpatients, elective patients, day patients and acutely admitted patients.

Evidence for Specific Prevention

Specific prevention concerns prevention activities addressing specific groups of patients. Patient education and rehabilitation programmes are examples of this. Rehabilitation programmes that aim to support the individual's own ability to manage disease are thus part of the clinical guidelines for several patient groups, not as a supplementary aspect, but as part of treatment. The various education and rehabilitation programmes include common elements, e.g. counselling on smoking cessation, stopping or reducing alcohol intake, physical activity, nutrition, psychosocial support, patient education and optimizing the medical (or surgical or psychiatric) treatment.

Heart Patients

Ischaemic heart disease is one of the biggest disease groups in the hospital sector and is the source of large, and ever increasing, pressure of demand on the health care sector altogether. Formerly rehabilitation of heart patients primarily concerned physical training, but against the background of the scientific results achieved over the past 10 to 15 years, the concept of heart rehabilitation has been extended to cover the following elements:

- physical training;

- lifestyle intervention and risk factor control: support to change of eating habits, smoking cessation, alcohol reduction, moderate physical training and preventive medical treatment;
- patient education;
- psychosocial care;
- medical treatment of symptoms;
- systematic control and follow up.

Results from international, controlled studies show evidence that heart rehabilitation may provide significant health outcomes in the form of:

- reduction of the number of admissions, both readmissions and overall cardiac admissions;
- maintenance of the patient's functional level;
- improvement of the patient's health related quality of life;
- improvement of overall risk factor control through lifestyle change and enhanced medical compliance.

There is a high level of evidence for the value of cardiac rehabilitation.

Chronic Lung Patients

Chronic obstructive lung disease (COPD) is a frequently occurring disease and is the cause of 20 to 25 % of admissions to medical departments in Europe. COPD is one of the five most resource demanding diseases in Denmark. Over the past 20 years many different lung rehabilitation programmes have been developed and tested, and there is now documentation that these programmes lead to:

- alleviation of breathing difficulty;
- increase in the distance that the patient is able to walk;
- improved physical capacity;
- improved functional level in everyday life;
- improved quality of life;
- improved ability to cope with disease and aggravation of disease;
- fewer admissions.

It is still not clear what the optimum structure, content and duration of COPD rehabilitation programmes is, however, there is agreement that as a minimum the following elements should be included:

- smoking cessation assistance;

- physical training/training in the home;
- physiotherapy;
- nutritional counselling;
- psychosocial support;
- patient education.

There is a moderate to high level of evidence for the value of rehabilitation after lung disease.

Asthma Patients

Asthma is a widespread disease, which occurs in about 5% of the adult population and in 5 to 10% of school children in most European countries. Over the past 30 to 40 years, a large number of randomized studies have been carried out in order to throw light on the effect of various education programmes. The programmes have been tested both in the hospital sector and in general practice. The resulting evidence has been summarized in several reviews and a Cochrane study, which conclude that there is documentation that patients who take part in asthma education programmes focusing on the training of skills achieve considerable effects, such as:

- fewer admissions;
- less absence from work;
- fewer asthma attacks at night;
- improvement of the patient's general capacity;
- improved medical compliance;
- improved quality of life.

It is still not clear what the optimum structure, content and duration of education programmes for asthma patients is. Usually programmes cover 4 to 5 lessons in the course of a couple of weeks.

There is a high level of evidence for the value of rehabilitation among asthma patients.

Diabetes Patients

Type 1-diabetes occurs in all age groups. Less is known about the occurrence of type 2-diabetes than about type 1-diabetes. The occurrence of type 2-diabetes is increasing rapidly and because of the increase in overweight/obesity it is seen in younger and younger persons. With regard to both types of diabetes the most significant health risk is development of late complications (risk of cardiovascular disease increased 3 to 5 times) and occurrence of diabetic eye disease, renal disorder and nervous disorder (retinopathy, nephropathy and neuropathy).

A number of randomized and controlled studies have been carried out with regard to both type 1 and type 2 diabetes. These studies all show that interventions with regard to one or several risk factors that can lead to late complications are effective.

Interventions should address:

- near normalization of blood sugar;
- near normalization of blood pressure and blood fat levels;
- smoking cessation;
- psychosocial support;
- counselling on nutrition, including alcohol, and physical activity.

There is a high level of evidence for the value of diabetic rehabilitation.

Osteoporosis Patients

There is an increase in the prevalence of osteoporosis in the western world, among other things because of an increase in the number of elderly persons. The risk of osteoporosis-related fractures increases considerably with age and is especially frequent in women. The three most frequent osteoporosis-related fractures occur in different age groups. Fracture in or near the wrist increases markedly from the age of 55, back problems from the age of 65, and fracture in or around the hip from the age of 75.

There is evidence that increased calcium intake in childhood may increase bone mineral content. There is no agreement as to whether women may benefit from calcium intake after the menopause. But there are studies that indicate that calcium intake along with vitamin D, reduce the number of fractures in elderly men and women. Physical activity and an active lifestyle increase bone mineral content along with enhanced muscle strength and muscle coordination, which contributes to reduction of the risk of fractures. Smoking increases the risk of osteoporosis in women because female smokers have an earlier menopause than non-smokers and enhanced oestradiol metabolism. In the same way alcohol abuse in men constitutes a significant risk factor for the development of osteoporosis because of poor nutrition and reduced testosterone production.

Thus primary prevention should address:

- smoking cessation;

- reduction or cessation of alcohol consumption;
- motivation for physical activity.

Furthermore there is evidence that hip protectors reduce the number of fractures by 67% among elderly persons in rest homes. Thus hip protectors are an important element of the prevention programmes for frail elderly persons who are prone to falls and osteoporosis.

There is a low to moderate high level of evidence for rehabilitation among these patients.

Patients with Cancer

A reduction of the occurrence of cancer is a primary goal in health care plans in most countries whereas rehabilitation of cancer patients has not been considered equally. It is estimated that two thirds of newly diagnosed cancer patients need rehabilitation services.

It is necessary to initiate further knowledge in this area, however interventions should address:

- psychosocial support and counselling;
- physical training/relaxation;
- nutrition guidance;
- smoking cessation;
- sexual problems;
- communication of knowledge to patients and relatives.

There is a low level of evidence for cancer rehabilitation.

Stroke

Stroke is a serious condition in so far as 40% of the patients die during the first year after onset of the disease, and many patients are not able to return to their own homes.

Many factors increase the risk of stroke: smoking, alcohol abuse, lack of physical activity, increased blood fat levels, hypertension, diabetes, irregular heartbeat. The risk increases with age. There is evidence that patients participating in rehabilitation in the form of comprehensive interdisciplinary treatment through all the phases of the disease may achieve:

- a reduction of mortality of 25%-50%;
- a reduced need for residential homes of 40%;
- improved functional level.

Furthermore prevention includes counselling on smoking cessation, stop drinking or reduction of alcohol consumption, regulation of blood fat levels, optimization of blood pressure and heart function as well as anticoagulant therapy. Thus, it is recommended that patients with stroke are admitted to special stroke units where rehabilitation may be initiated already in the acute phase.

There is a high level of evidence for rehabilitation after apoplexy.

Patients with Psychiatric Disorders

A large proportion of psychiatric patients is smokers or have other substance abuse problems. Treatment with psychoactive medicine leads to considerable weight gain in many patients and therefore there is a need for intervention with regard to nutrition and physical activity. Physical activity in psychiatric patients has a documented positive effect on the course of treatment. Thus, prevention should be integrated in psychiatric patient pathways in the same way as in somatic pathways.

Work has been carried out concerning documentation and evaluation of various ways of organizing treatment, e.g. in the form of Assertive Community Treatment teams. There is evidence that Assertive Community Treatment Teams that address patients with a large use of inpatient days may reduce the cost of hospital treatment, increase the number who are in contact with the treatment system, and improve user satisfaction among patients and relatives. There is also a positive effect with regard to a number of social parameters, e.g. homelessness or not having an independent home. It is recommended that outreach psychosis teams be introduced generally for the treatment of patients with long-term psychotic disorders.

There is a high to moderate level of evidence for psychiatric rehabilitation.

Surgical Patients

A varying number of patients that undergo surgical intervention suffer from long-term and complicated conditions. The development of complications can be related to the diagnosis and the spread of the disease, type of intervention and the organization, i.e. staff competence, use of clinical guidelines etc. In recent years, we have acquired new knowledge on the significance of the patient's general lifestyle habits with regard to tobacco, alcohol, nutrition and exercise in connection with intervention. There is now evidence that targeted prevention initiatives can reduce the number of complications. The significance of increased risk of complications due to the above mentioned factors should form part of overall indications for surgery. As in the case of intervention with regard to medical patients with chronic disorders, qualitative intervention should comprise seven elements, i.e. tobacco, alcohol, physical activity, nutrition, psychosocial support, medical (including surgical and anaesthetic) optimization and patient education.

Against the backdrop of available evidence, the National Board of Health has established general recommendations for intervention with regard to tobacco and alcohol in connection with surgical intervention. Early mobilization and nutrition have been described as significant elements of the postoperative phase.

Smoking

Altogether smokers have three times as many complications in the form of poor healing of wounds and other tissue and heart and lung complications in connection with surgical intervention compared to non-smokers.

Alcohol

Excessive alcohol consumption is linked to increased surgical risk, which increases with consumption so that there are three times as many complications in patients who consume five or more units per day. Complications are due to alcohol-induced organ damage that is reversible to a wide extent if no alcohol is consumed.

Nutrition

There is evidence that nutritional intervention for undernourished patients reduces complications in connection with surgical intervention by 10% and reduces the frequency of infection and increases muscle strength in surgical patients. There is also evidence that resumption of food intake immediately after intervention considerably reduces complications.

Physical Activity

Early mobilization and increased physical activity following surgery has turned out to be significant and is part of a new overall concept for rehabilitation in connection with surgery. The intervention reduces weight loss and the fatigue often seen after surgery.

Preventive intervention that should be offered systematically:

- identification of risk factors;
- dialogue with the patient to clarify the role of these factors and the patients' own responsibility and options for influencing their own situation;
- evidence-based offer of intervention and follow up.

Intervention with regard to surgical patients is supported by the high motivation for changes in lifestyle prior to surgery, as measured by surprisingly high compliance. Patient information should include the high postoperative morbidity related to lifestyle factors, and the evidence based programme should be offered in due time before surgery.

PATIENTS FOR HEALTH PROMOTING SELF CARE IN HOSPITALS

Even if patients are not only understood as the object of treatment but also as coproducers of their health outcomes, we have to take into account that they can only fulfil their patient role in relation to the trinity of body, psyche, social status). Depending on their condition, the patient's contribution to co-production ranges selfcare of the patient, over professionally supported care to intensive care (heart/lung machine). Following the four criteria of the complex concept of health gain, reproduction concerns all three dimensions of health – the physical (e.g. adequate nutrition), the mental (e.g. enough privacy in the hospital), and the social (e.g. possibilities for contacts with relatives, patient support).

In order to avoid hospitalization as far as possible, it should be made a principle to allow for as much selfcare as possible, and to provide as much professional care as necessary. To make selfcare possible under the difficult conditions of partly severely ill individuals outside their usual household environment, and subjected to the bureaucratic imperatives of the hospital organization, professional care has to be as empowering as possible, and needs to take into account cultural differences of patients. Empowerment again includes physical, mental and social dimensions, knowledge, skills and motivations. This again can be seen as the specific contribution of health promotion.

The effects of this strategy have not been systematically researched, but examples of interventions that have been successfully implemented in specific hospitals are:

- visiting and lay support services to support the psychosocial needs of patients;

- patient information about general hospital features (e.g. where to find what; visiting hours) at hospital admission;
- offers and options to encourage patient activities and patient self-responsibility (e.g. exercise, culture activities, patient libraries, discussions, patient internet cafe);
- provide psychological assistance to cope with stress or anxieties related to the hospital stay or to the patient's disease (e.g. cancer).

Co-production in Treatment and Care

The core task of the modern acute care hospital is to offer diagnostic and therapeutic services for incidents of acute illness (of a rather severe type or with the need/opportunity for technical diagnostics and treatment) as well as acute episodes of chronic disease – for inpatients and outpatients.

The second health promotion strategy relates to the long and changing tradition of quality assurance and quality improvement of core tasks – starting with the education of professionals, and in the last 20 years switching towards developing processes and structures of organizations and larger systems. How can health promotion contribute to the quality improvement of core processes in hospitals?

The concept of empowerment stresses the necessity that individuals take control over their health – which means in the context of the hospital that patients are not only seen as objects of interventions but also as co-producers of these interventions – an idea that fits well with other traditions of analysing services as co-produced. As the co-producer has to actively contribute to the process, he/she has to be actively empowered for making this contribution. This sort of empowerment cannot be achieved by the clinical/technical interventions themselves, but by communicative/educative interventions. Medicine has to open itself towards education. Education refers to the transfer of knowledge (data, information), training of skills and enhancement of motivation.

The concept of health gain defines the relevant output of the hospital interventions in a more complex way: clinical outcome + quality of life + patient satisfaction + health literacy. These outcomes refer to all three aspects of health: physical, mental and social. The treatment process itself has to become more complex. The focus stays on effective treatment, but in order to optimize health gain, aspects of disease prevention, health protection and health development have to get due attention within treatment (systematically avoid risks, use opportunities to build health resources – biological, mental, social).

A practical example for empowering patients for co-production would be diagnosisand treatment related patient information, training and counselling (e.g. by informing patients about how they can contribute to the recuperation process; by describing alternatives and side effects), in order to enable patients to participate in the diagnostic process (e.g. by providing all information needed); participate in treatment-related decision-making; participate in treatment and care processes (e.g. by complying with the prescriptions).

There is clear evidence that this type of patient empowerment can, e.g. for surgical patients, reduce post-surgical complications, and can speed up recovery. Development of the Hospital into a supportive, health promoting and empowering setting for patients.

The hospital does not only consist of service processes, but also of a context within which the services are provided. Just like the services produce (health) outputs/outcomes, the context/situation/setting has impacts that are relevant for health.

There are impacts of the material setting (hospital infections, quality of air, temperature, sick building syndrome etc.) and also impacts of the hospital as a social setting with its organizational structure and culture, that influence opportunities for coproduction and selfcare of patients and of course the professional treatment and care for patients. What is the contribution of HP for settings development? Health promotion pays specific attention to supportive environments – physical as well as social, and enlarges the focus on results from clinical outcomes also to other dimensions of health gain.

GROWTH AND DEVELOPMENT OF THE TODDLER

Toddlers are children who are 1 to 2 years of age. This time period is a stage of growth for young child. During this time, he will go through many changes in his physical, psychological (mental and emotional), and social development.

Features

The most visible signs of a toddler's normal growth are the physical changes. Weight and length gradually increase. The muscles start to develop, enabling full control of his movements. Sitting without the help of an adult and taking the first steps are also part of the normal development of a toddler. Picking up toys and turning the pages of storybooks can also be demonstrated at this period.

First words are soon uttered, and he will associate pictures with words—both signs that communication skills are developing normally. Emotional and social development during the toddler years starts to show when the child forms an attachment to his caregiver. He also starts to throw tantrums and experience quick mood changes.

Factors Affecting a Toddler's Development

Some factors affect the normalcy of the toddler years. Eating habits, especially if a toddler demonstrates lack of appetite or is picky in selecting food, can affect growth. Problems affecting his health such as poor eyesight or difficulty in hearing can be hindrances, too. Play is also integral to normal development, as is sleep. Sleep lets babies grow. Lack of sleep creates behaviour problems that can inhibit development.

Effects

The importance of having normal toddler years leads to the next successful growth stages of a child. From birth to the toddler years, modern medical science has paved the way for detecting future illnesses or inherent diseases. If toddler doesn't encounter setbacks at this time and all signs of normal behaviour are assessed, the rest of his childhood will be almost always normal.

Considerations

Parents can promote normal growth in toddlers by taking a proactive role in communication. Reading books to toddlers further develops their speech and reading skills. Playing helps form a bond between parent and child but also enhances creativity. Proper nutrition and sleep should be followed. Light disciplinary measures can be given to curb tantrums and bad behaviour.

Physical changes occur during the toddler years

Child's body grows and changes as he learns to do new things.

Movement

Child's muscles develop as his motor (movement) skills get better.

Body Control or Movement

Child may sit without support at about one year of age. He may start walking on his own or still need to hold hand. Later, he may be able to jump.

Hand and Finger Control

Child learns to use his hands. He may be able to hold a book without help and turn board pages, which are thicker than regular pages.

Weight and Length

Child may gain four times his birth weight during this time. His length may increase to about 22 inches. The length of child's height measured while he is lying down.

Changes in communication occur during the toddler years

Childs becomes interested in his environment. His language skills improve as he tries to let others know his thoughts.

Speech

Childs tries to form words, which may result to babbling (talking without meaning) at first. Later, he learns to use actions to tell what he wants. He learns a lot of words, which may start to come out like sentences. At around two years of age, he may be able to make 2 to 3 word sentences.

Understanding Words

Child may be able to point to a body part when named or point to pictures in books. Later, he may be able to name familiar pictures. He may recite or fill in words in stories that he knows. Child may also be able to follow simple directions and requests.

Emotional and social changes occur during the toddler years

Child starts to express his feelings and interact with other people.

Attachment and Tears

During the toddler years, Child wants to be near his caregiver. A caregiver may be the child's parent, relative, or babysitter. Child will not like to be away from his caregiver or around strangers. He may play beside other children, but may not want to play or share toys with them. Child may be anxious around objects that he is not familiar with. He may fear heights and may even be afraid of the toilet.

Behaviour

Child wants to be in control and may insist on doing things himself.

He may seem stubborn, refuse help, and get easily frustrated. He may often say "no"' when he is asked a question. His mood may easily change and lead to temper tantrums.

Factors may affect a toddler's development

Certain medical Conditions

Problems that affect hearing or the brain may also slow child's ability to speak well. These problems may include infections and head injuries.

Eating Habits

Toddlers often become picky of what they eat and may prefer certain foods. Refusing to eat, or only eating fast food or junk food may decrease child's growth and development.

Play

Playing helps a child develop his imagination. Child will also learn how to get along with others.

Sleep

Child needs sleep to grow and develop normally. The total time spent sleeping includes naps in the morning and afternoon, and sleep without waking up at night. Lack of sleep decreases child's energy. Daytime behaviour is worse if child is a poor sleeper. If child does not have enough naps during the day, it is important that he sleeps more at night.

Help of child during his toddler years

- As child starts to speak, learn the signs or actions he uses in place of words. Be patient and give child time to finish his thought. Try to understand what he is saying. Do not use complex or very simple sentences when talking to him. Speaking to child using clear sentences will help him learn how to communicate better.
- Give child a variety of healthy foods each day. This should include fruit, vegetables, bread products, dairy products, and protein (such as chicken, fish and beans). Have child sit with the family at mealtime even if he does not like to eat. This way, he will still see different foods and develop his taste at his own pace. Do not force child to eat. You may need to offer him a food 10 or more times before he eats it. Give him healthy snacks between meals, and water to drink.

- Make sure to keep regular appointments with child's caregivers for check-ups and vaccinations.
- Make sure child gets enough sleep (about 12 to 14 hours) every night. Schedule his sleep with the same bed time and wake time each day. Bedtime routines are also helpful for child. Do not place a television in child's room, and keep the room cool and dark.
- Play with child. This helps his learning, boosts his self-confidence, and improves his skills. Store toys or objects that may cause choking, poisoning, or other accidents away from child. Store toys when he is not using them. Computer and video games should only be used with an adult. These should be used for 1 to 2 hours a day or less. All games should be fit to child's age.
- Read with child. This helps develop his language and reading skills. Place books fit for his age within his reach.
- Time out may be used as a way to discipline toddler. This lets him quiet down and think about what he did. It also gives time to calm down and stay in control. Set limits for child. Praise and reward child when it is suitable. Do not criticize or show disapproval of child when he has done something wrong. Explain what you would like him to do instead, and tell him why toddler continues to grow steadily. However, after the 2nd birthday, growth slows. By age 2, toddler weighs four times his or her birth weight, usually measures about 34 inches in length, and has a head size that has grown to almost 90 per cent of adult head size.

Between the 2nd and 3rd birthdays, toddler will usually put on only 3-5 pounds and add only about 3 inches in length. During the toddler years, the soft, round look of baby changes. Baby fat begins to disappear from cheeks, arms and legs. Child develops a neck. Muscles "bulk up" as muscle mass increases twice as fast as bone. Legs are longer and straighter and feet point forward. 1-year-old's flat feet develop arches as the fat pad that hid the arch disappears.

Brain Fact

During the toddler years, amazing changes are taking place in the brain. The brain is growing in complexity as the number of connections between nerve cells increases to 1,000 trillion, which is twice the number of connections at birth (and twice the number in an adult brain). In addition, there are three other changes. The supporting cells of the brain multiply. Individual nerves are insulated for more efficient firing, and new blood vessels are formed to supply areas of increased activity with oxygen and nutrients.

Dental Development

By age 2-1/2, most children have all 20 of their baby or primary teeth. The second molars are the last to appear usually coming in between 20 and 30 months.

Child's primary teeth are important for chewing, speaking, and child's smile. Primary teeth are also important for jaw growth. They hold a place for permanent teeth.

Sixty per cent of 3-year-olds have one or more cavities. One of the most important things you can do for child's smile is to take good care of baby's teeth – regular tooth brushing, a healthy diet, a minimum of sticky, sugary foods and regular visits to the dentist beginning at age 12-18 months.

Milestones: Physical Skills

Usually around 18 months, child is practicing physical skills every waking hour. You'll be amazed at child's progress with coordination and balance. Some highlights include walking backwards, walking up stairs holding someone's hand, being able to bend over to pick up a toy, and being able to remove larger pieces of clothing.

Usually around 24 months, child can walk up and down stairs alone and may want to try jumping off the bottom step. Child can also use a spoon well, kick a large ball, build a tower of six blocks, and unzip a zipper.

Usually around 36 months, child can walk up and down steps alternating feet, can open a door by turning a knob, can bend over easily without falling, and can ride a large wheeled toy like a tricycle. At this age, child's favourite activity may be running. Get ready!

Useful Info: Living with an Intense Toddler

Toddler years are especially challenging for children with intense temperaments. Try these techniques to make life easier for child (and for you). If child is: Intensely active: Schedule lots of supervised active play in safe spaces – outside whenever possible. Intensely loud: Ask child to save loud noises for outdoors and use an "inside voice" when indoors. Encourage singing and reciting nursery rhymes.

Play Activities

How? Tell the child to copy movements. Point to ear saying, "Daddy says point to ear." Child should imitate you. Try pointing to nose and then toes, each time saying, "Daddy says point to nose" or "Daddy says point to toes." Throw in a few "Daddy says stick out tongue" or "Daddy says make a funny face" just so you can get toddler giggling. Don't expect the game to last for more than a few minutes.

Why? Toddlers love to imitate, they love activity, and they love having fun, but they have very short attention spans.

Baby may need a developmental evaluation if by his or her 3rd birthday, he or she:

- Falls frequently and has difficulty with stairs.
- Drools or has speech that is difficult to understand.
- Has difficulty handling small objects.
- Cannot copy a circle.
- Doesn't understand simple instructions.
- Is not interested or has very little interest in other children.
- Does not have pretend play.
- Does not put two words together.
- Is unable to separate from parents without significant protest.

Child is able to solve problems by thinking and doing. toddler can recognize same and different and begins to have more complicated play. In addition being able to sort objects by colour and shape, child understands the idea of numbers, especially two.

Toddler years are a time of magical thinking when child finds it difficult to separate fantasy from reality. Magical thinking can be delightful, for example, a visit from an imaginary friend. It can also be dangerous, for example, a 2-1/2 year old deciding to fly down the steps like Superman.

Books for Toddler

Reading books to toddler does more than provide entertainment. Sharing books together provides a message that books are important. Reading is a crucial skill for success in school. Help child get a head start by starting early.

Toddler is interested in books if he or she brings you a book to read, tries to hold the book, wants to turn the pages, points at the pictures, asks for the same story over and over, carries a book around the house, or sits and "reads" a book out loud.

Major Milestones: Language

Mastery of speech and language is perhaps the most variable of developmental milestones. About 1 in every 10 to 15 children has some difficulty with language or speech. Try to be both watchful and reasonable with expectations. It helps to know that boys usually talk later than girls. Share any concerns you might have with child's doctor.

Toddler is better at understanding language than producing it. Children can point to a body part before they can name it. Some of the most important milestones of the toddler years are imitates animal sounds; refers to self by name; begins to use "I" and "me;" begins to combine words in 2- and 3-word sentences; uses "please" and "thank you;" adds "ed" to verbs to indicate past tense like "I walked" and "s" to nouns to indicate plurals like "dogs;" asks what, where, when and why questions; uses 4 and 5 words in sentences; can be mostly understood by strangers; and understands "on," "in," and "under."

A continuing theme in child's development is the relationship between attachment and achievement. In the first year, child's eagerness to explore depends on child's sense of security. In the toddler years, child's ability to learn depends on feeling secure.

The importance of attachment doesn't go away. In school-age years, children of equal intelligence are most likely to achieve in schoolwork if they have a strong parent-child attachment.

Emotional Development

Toddlers are incredibly self-centered. You may observe a few of these behaviors: refusing to share, temper tantrums, biting or hitting.

Most toddlers are intense at least part of the time. They can be extremely happy, extremely sad, and extremely angry all within 15 minutes. If child's temperament is intense, you're likely to see temper tantrums. If child is quiet, you may see clinginess or whining. It's all part of the same developmental process. Child is trying to work out how to behave around others. Soothing ruffled feelings and calming angry tantrums is a huge plus for child's development.

By the time child reaches 3 years, he or she is able to take turns in games, show affection for playmates, understand "mine" and "his" and "hers," and show more self-control. child also begins to show concern for others.

Child becomes more aware of pleasing or displeasing you during the toddler years. Somewhere around 3, toddlers show emotions such as shame, embarrassment, pride, guilt, and even envy. Self-awareness is a major emotional milestone. Now child knows that you have expectations and knows whether he or she is living up to them. This is the first step toward the development of conscience.

Child Rearing Myth

Parents who childproof their homes and who constantly watch their toddlers are being overprotective. Children should learn the rules.

Child Rearing Fact

Toddlers are too young to be expected to remember and follow the rules. Since toddlers don't have the knowledge or experience to avoid danger or keep their hands off breakables, they require constant watching – especially in a home that hasn't been childproofed.

Keep a bottle of syrup of ipecac (non-prescription – costs about 2) on hand and locked in first-aid kit. Use only on direction of doctor or the Indiana Poison Centre. Toddlers are curious. They put everything in their mouths. It's no wonder that 1- to 3-year-olds are at the greatest risk for poisoning. Now that child can climb, open doors and drawers, and open bottles, everything that could be harmful must be out of sight and out of reach.

Guardian Angel

If there is one time in childhood child requires a guardian angel, it's the toddler years. Toddlers need constant protection. Be especially watchful when children are hungry, for example, before mealtimes and in the late afternoon. At times of stress or confusion like holidays, family illness, houseguests, or moving day, children are at an increased risk of injury or harm and need extra protection.

Health Alert: To Grand mother's House We Go

Attention all grandparents. Be sure to enroll in a CPR and first-aid course as soon as you know you'll be grandparents. Prepare carefully for a visit from newly walking grandchild – as well as older toddlers and preschoolers. Use the "Room-by-Room Checklist" in the Child Safety section to childproof any rooms that will not be kept locked during grandchild's visit. More than one-third of all poisonings occur in the homes of children's grandparents. Toddlers will eat anything. Since you can't guard against all the dangers grandchildren can find, you'll need to take turn as a guardian angel watching over little ones.

GROWTH AND DEVELOPMENT OF THE PRESCHOOLER

Three and four-year-old children are often called preschoolers. Preschool children are making developmental strides and express an interest in the world around them. They want to touch, taste, smell, hear, and test things for themselves. They are eager to learn. They learn by experiencing and by doing. Preschoolers learn from their play. They are busy developing skills, using language, and struggling to gain inner control. Preschoolers want to establish themselves as separate from their parents. They are more independent than toddlers. They can express their needs since they have greater command of lan-guage.

Fears often develop during the preschool years. Common fears include new places and experiences and separation from parents and other important people. You can expect the preschool child to test over and over again, to use profanity and other forbidden words, and to act very silly. Preschoolers may still have trouble getting along with other children, and sharing may still be difficult. Because of their developing imaginations and rich fantasy lives, they may have trouble telling fantasy from reality. They may also talk about imaginary friends. Preschoolers need clear and simple rules so that they know the boundaries of acceptable behaviour.

Understanding their growth and development will help you guide preschoolers through this stage. This fact sheet lists some of the characteristics of preschoolers. These characteristics are listed for three main areas: physical (body), social (getting along with others) and emotional (feelings), and intellectual (thinking and language) development. Remember that all preschoolers are different and reach the various stages at different times.

Preschoolers are children who are 2 to 5 years of age. This time period is a stage of continuing growth and development for young child. He will go through many changes in his physical, mental, emotional and social development.

Preschooler's body "makeover" begins at the top and works down. The bones of the skull and face grow so that child's face loses some of its roundness, and child develops a more noticeable forehead, nose and chin. Meanwhile, the upper and lower jaws widen to make room for permanent teeth. The padded shoulder "football player" look of the toddler changes, too. child's shoulders narrow, posture improves, and that "toddler tummy" flattens.

Child's requirement for dietary fat decreases in the preschool years. As preschooler's body matures, it's time to cut down on high-fat foods like whole milk and cheese. The low-fat diet that is good for you is now good for child.

Sleep Disturbances

There are several normal sleep behaviors beginning in the preschool years that can be very worrisome to parents:

Sleep Terrors: Sleep terrors, also called night terrors, may begin as young as age 2. Sleep terrors differ from nightmares. Nightmares are frightening dreams during dream sleep and can be remembered upon awaking. Sleep terrors occur in non-dream sleep and cannot be remembered upon awaking. They usually occur 1 to 4 hours after falling asleep and last between 5 and 30 minutes. They may occur several times in one night or only once in a lifetime. Sleep terrors are far worse for the parents than for the child.

Typically, the child appears to be awake, screams, cries, may thrash, and looks very frightened. Because the child is not fully awake, the child cannot be calmed. When the episode ends, the child returns to full sleep. The good news is children outgrow sleep terrors.

The best way to handle sleep terrors is to stay with child so that you can protect him or her from any injury caused by thrashing movements. Don't turn on the lights or try to wake child. Child will have no memory of the episode. It may help to put child to bed earlier in case being overtired is contributing to the problem. If the night terrors are very frequent, discuss the problem with doctor.

Sleep Talking: Sleep talking includes talking, laughing, and crying out in sleep. Child is not aware of what is going on. Even if child answers questions, he or she will have no memory of the conversation. Sleep talking is so common it is not considered abnormal.

Sleep Walking: Sleep walking may involve only walking or may include a number of other activities, including dressing, raiding the refrigerator, opening doors, and even going up and down stairs. As with night terrors, don't try to wake child. Gently guide child back to bed and feel better knowing child will have no memory of this in the morning.

Milestones: Physical Skills

Usually around the age of 3, child becomes much more coordinated when running or going up and down the stairs. By the end of the preschool years, child can catch a bounced ball most of the time, kick a ball forward, and stand on one foot or hop. Three-year-olds are so active that sometimes they find it easier to substitute a movement for a word. They may run around the room with their arms spread out to indicate flying instead of talking about flying.

Handedness is well established by age 3. If child prefers to use his or her left hand, don't try to change it. Lefties do just fine.

Child's ability to concentrate allows child to take advantage of the gains in small muscle control in his or her hands. child's is able to copy a circle and to scribble quite happily. When playing with blocks, Child can build a tower of nine or more cubes.

This is a great age for crafts. Child loves to practice cutting, painting, and coloring. For future gardeners, it's a great time to work in the garden. For future carpenters, nothing beats the thrill of using a real screwdriver.

Self-help skills are much improved. At this age, children can feed themselves, unbutton their clothes, and handle large zippers and snaps.

Play Activities!

How? Find three pictures that show something happening like a boy riding a bike, falling off, and his mother coming to him. Paste the pictures on to 3 × 5 cards. Ask child what happened first, next, and last.

Why? Practicing placing cards in an order that makes sense will help child at school.

Preschooler may need a developmental evaluation if, as the 5th birthday nears, he or she:

- Has difficulty throwing a ball overhand
- Is unable to jump in place
- Is unable to hold a crayon correctly
- Is unable to stack four blocks
- Won't separate willingly from parents
- Is not interested in other children

- Is not interested in interactive games
- Responds very little to non-family members
- Has no imaginative play
- Is uncooperative with dressing, sleeping, toilet training
- Has difficulty with self-control when angered or upset
- Is unable to give his or her first and last name
- Does not use plurals or past tense properly
- Does not use "me" and "you" correctly
- Does not speak in sentences of more than three words
- Seems unhappy or sad most of the time

Learning/Thinking

Preschoolers continue to use magical thinking to solve problems or explain things. You'll be surprised what you learn when you ask child a "why?" question. For example, preschooler may tell you that the sun comes up in the morning because that is when it wakes up.

Sometimes an answer alerts you to a possible problem, such as child believing that his or her anger could make someone ill. Be firm when you explain that emotions don't cause illness or harm to others.

Preschoolers are not logical thinkers. They believe what their eyes tell them even if it makes no sense. Try this famous experiment with preschooler to get a better understanding of how child thinks. Pour water from a tall, thin glass vase into a wide, clear glass bowl. Make sure no water spills. Ask preschooler which container has more water. Very likely, child will answer the tall, thin vase (or whichever container appears larger to the child). It's unlikely that preschooler will say that the amount of water has not changed and it only looks different.

Even if you point out that no water was added or taken away, preschooler believes what he or she can see and pays no attention to logic. This is called prelogical thinking and is absolutely normal and charming.

Stuttering

One of the common concerns of parents of preschoolers is stuttering. About 1 in 20 children in this age group stutters. Boys are troubled more than girls. Children tend to stutter when they are tired, upset or talking quickly. Stuttering may actually be an unconscious way for child to hold a space in the conversation until he or she can get the word or sentence out.

Don't call attention to stuttering. Ignore it. Most stuttering goes away on its own, usually within two to three months. If child's stutters, it might help if you talk slower or make a point of sitting down when child talks to you so that child's will not feel hurried. Warning signs that child's stuttering is not likely to be outgrown include child feeling very self-conscious about stuttering; losing eye contact with the person to whom he or she is speaking while stuttering; frequently repeating words or parts of words; having facial twitches; breathing faster or showing other signs of difficulty in forming words; stuttering for more than six months; or having a family history of a parent or sibling with stuttering problems.

If child's stuttering is causing behaviour or emotional problems or any of the above warning signs are present, discuss the problem with doctor.

GROWTH AND DEVELOPMENT OF THE SCHOOL-AGE CHILD

The middle to late school age years are a time of great change in child's. In addition to starting puberty, his mind will also grow to understand logical and abstract thinking and he will develop the moral standards by which he will live his life. You can also expect him to begin to move away from the family as he develops his own identity and also become more influenced by his friends. Fortunately, this influence is usually limited to outward things, such as hair and clothing styles.

This is a time of growing independence and children at this age want to be considered more responsible. To help foster this sense of responsibility, now is a good time to begin giving child an allowance. The amount is not very important, but is usually 50 cents to 1.00 per year in age and should be used for special things that child wants. Managing an allowance will help to teach child about the value of money and the importance of saving.

While it is also important that child begin to have regular age appropriate chores (setting or clearing the table, taking out the garbage, cleaning their room, etc.) around the house, these should probably not be tied to his allowance. Positive reinforcement is important for completed chores, and failure to complete chores can be punished by loss of a privilege (TV, videogames, etc.). Allowing child to have a choice of which chore to do sometimes helps with compliance.

Encourage self esteem and a positive self image in child by using positive reinforcement and frequent praise for things that he has accomplished. Encourage child to be curious, explore and take on new challenges. Also be sure to prepare child for puberty and sexual development and begin sexuality education if you have not already done so, including that abstinence is the safest way to prevent pregnancy and sexually transmitted diseases.

School Age Healthy Habits

Regularly talk to child's about the proper habits that can help him lead a healthy life. These include getting proper nutrition (eating three meals a day and two nutritious snacks, limiting high sugar and high fat foods, eating fruits, vegetables, lean meats and low fat dairy products, including 3 servings of milk, cheese or yogurt to meet his calcium needs), regular exercise, adequate sleep (nine hours each night), and participation in extracurricular activities at school and in the community. Begin preparing child for their plans after graduation.

It is also very important to begin communicating with child to help prevent him from picking up bad habits, including the use of tobacco, alcohol and drugs (including the use of inhalants; especially aerosols and glue; and newer drugs like GHB and Ecstasy which many kids think are safe). Children whose parents talk to them regularly are at much less risk for experimenting with cigarettes, alcohol and drugs. Teach them how to avoid situations where drugs, alcohol, or cigarettes are present and to choose friends who also choose not to use these substances.

Emphasize to them that these substances can hurt him, can make him sick, can cause decreased lung function and problems playing sports, and that it is OK to say no. Also, do not let him attend parties that are unsupervised by adults and let him know that he can communicate openly with you about these difficult subjects. Watch for the warning signs of drug use, including a sudden change in his behaviour or personality, decreased performance in school, or changes in which friends he associates with.

While all children may grow at a different rate, the following indicates the average for school-aged children 6 to 12 years old:

- *Weight*: Average gain of about 5 to 7 pounds a year
- *Height*: Average growth of about 2.5 inches per year

What can Child do at This Age?

As child's continues to grow, you will notice new and exciting abilities that child develops. While children may progress at different rates and have diverse interests, the following are some of the common milestones children may reach in this age group:

- 6- to 7-year-olds:
  - Enjoys many activities and stays busy
  - Likes to paint and draw
  - May lose first tooth
  - Vision is as sharp as an adult's vision
  - Practices skills in order to become better
  - Jumps rope
  - Rides a bike
- 8- to 9-year-olds:
  - More graceful with movements and abilities
  - Jumps, skips, and chases
  - Dresses and grooms self completely
  - Can use tools (i.e., hammer, screwdriver)
- 10- to 12-year-olds:
  - Remainder of adult teeth will develop
  - Likes to sew and paint

What does Childs understand?

As children enter into school-age, their abilities and understanding of concepts and the world around them continue to grow. While children may progress at different rates, the following are some of the common milestones children may reach in this age group:

- 6- to 7-year-olds:
  - Understands concept of numbers
  - Knows daytime and nighttime
  - Knows right and left hands
  - Can copy complex shapes, such as a diamond
  - Can tell time
  - can understand commands with three separate Instructions
  - Can explain objects and their use
  - Can repeat three numbers backwards
  - Can read age-appropriate books and/or materials
- 8- to 9-year-olds:>

- Can count backwards
- Knows the date
- Reads more and enjoys reading
- Understands fractions
- Understands concept of space
- Draws and paints
- Can name months and days of week, in order
- Enjoys collecting objects

• 10- to 12-year-olds:
- Writes stories
- Likes to write letters
- Reads well
- Enjoys using the telephone

How does Childs Interact with Others?

A very important part of growing up is the ability to interact and socialize with others. During the school-age years, parents will see a transition in their child as he/she moves from playing alone to having multiple friends and social groups. While friendships become more important, the child is still fond of his/her parents and likes being part of a family. While every child is unique and will develop different personalities, the following are some of the common behavioral traits that may be present in child:

• 6- to 7-year-olds:
- Cooperates and shares
- Will cheat, if able
- Jealous of others and siblings
- Likes to copy adults
- Likes to play alone, but friends are becoming Important
- Plays with friends of the same gender
- May have temper tantrums
- Modest about body
- Likes to play board games

• 8- to 9-year-olds:
- Likes competition and games

  - Starts to mix friends and play with children of the opposite gender
  - Modest about body
  - Enjoys clubs and groups, such as Boy Scouts or Girl Scouts
  - Becoming interested in boy-girl relationships, but does not admit it
- 10- to 12-year-olds:
  - Friends are very important; may have a best friend
  - Increased interest in the opposite gender
  - likes and respects parents
  - Enjoys talking to others

How to help increase school-aged child's social ability

Consider the following as ways to foster school-aged child's social abilities:

- Set and provide appropriate limits, guidelines, and expectations and consistently enforce using appropriate consequences.
- Model appropriate behaviour.
- Offer compliments for child being cooperative and for any personal achievements.
- Help child choose activities that are appropriate for child's abilities.
- Encourage child to talk with you and be open with his/her feelings.
- Encourage child to read and read with child.
- Encourage child to get involved with hobbies and other activities.
- Encourage physical activity.
- Encourage self-discipline; expect child to follow rules that are set.
- Teach child to respect and listen to authority figures.
- Encourage child to talk about peer pressure and help set guidelines to deal with peer pressure.
- Spend uninterrupted time together - giving full attention to child.
- Limit television, video, and computer time.

Growth and puberty

From 4 years of age until the onset of rapid growth in puberty (the adolescent growth spurt) the average rate of growth for boys and girls is about 5-6 cm/year. During this time the 'typical' boy is slightly taller than the 'typical' girl. This situation is temporarily reversed when girls reach their adolescent growth spurt at around 11 years old, some two years earlier than boys. At age 14 years, boys are near the peak of their growth spurt and overtake girls, whose growth spurt has nearly finished.

The difference in magnitude of these growth spurts largely explains the difference in final heights attained by boys compared with girls. Weight velocity is almost constant from age 3 to puberty (rising from an average of 2.0 to about 2.7 kg/year), since the increase in fat velocity balances the drop in velocity of muscular and skeletal dimensions. Body shape continues to change, since the rate of growth of some parts, such as the legs and arms, is greater than the rate of growth of others, such as the trunk.

The change is a steady one, a smoothly continuous development to the final prepubescent physique, rather than any passage through a series of separate stages.

At puberty, a very considerable change in growth rate occurs. There is a swift increase in body size, a change in shape and body composition, and a rapid development of the ovaries anteaters, the reproductive organs, and the characters signalling sexual maturity. Some of these changes are common to both sexes, but most are sex-specific. Some children grow slightly more slowly than others and reach puberty later than average.

They do, in the end, reach a normal height, though children who have short parents tend to be short themselves. At puberty, boys have a great increase in muscle size and strength, together with a series of physiological changes making them more capable than girls of doing heavy physical work, and running faster and longer.

The changes specifically adapt the male to his primitive primate role of hunting, fighting, and foraging. Such adolescent changes occur generally in primates, but are more marked in some species than in others. Man lies at about the middle of the primate range, in terms of both adolescent size increase and degree of sexual differentiation. During the adolescent growth spurt, for a year or more, the velocity of height increase approximately doubles; a boy is likely to be growing again at the rate he first experienced about age 2.

Practically all skeletal and muscular dimensions take part in the spurt, though not to an equal degree. Most of the spurt in height is due to acceleration of trunk length rather than length of legs. There is a fairly regular order in which the dimensions accelerate: leg length as a rule reaches its peak first, followed by trunk length and the body breadths, with shoulder width last amongst them. The earliest dimensions to reach their adult size are the head, hands, and feet. At adolescence, children, particularly girls, sometimes complain of having large hands and feet. They can be reassured that by the time they are fully grown their hands and feet will be a little smaller in proportion to their arms and legs, and considerably smaller in proportion to their trunk.

The adolescent growth spurt in skeletal and muscular dimension is closely related to the rapid development of the reproductive system, which takes place at this time.

In boys the first sign of puberty is usually an increase in the size of the testes and scrotum, with reddening and wrinkling of the scrotal skin. Slight growth of pubic hair may begin about the same time, but is usually a little later. The spurts in height and penile growth begin on average about a year after the first testicular acceleration. Axillary hair appears on average some two years after the beginning of pubic hair growth.

In boys, facial hair begins to grow at about the same as the axillary hair appears. Breaking of the voice occurs relatively late in adolescence, and is often a gradual process and so not suitable as a criterion of puberty.

In girls the appearance of the 'breast buds' is as a rule the first sign of puberty, though the appearance of pubic hair sometimes precedes it. The uterus and vagina develop simultaneously with the breasts. Menarche, the first menstrual period, is a late event in the sequence. It almost invariably occurs after the peak of the height spurt has been passed. Though it marks a definitive and probably mature stage of uterine development, it does not usually signify the attainment of full reproductive function. Early menstrual cycles may be more irregular than later ones, and often there is no ovulation. There is therefore frequently a period of adolescent sterility lasting a year to 18 months after menarche, but this cannot be relied upon in an individual case.

GROWTH AND DEVELOPMENT OF THE ADOLESCENT

The development of children ages 12 through 18 years old is expected to include predictable physical and mental milestones.

Adolescents are children who are 10 to 20 years of age. They are in a period between childhood and adulthood, called adolescence. This time period is divided into three stages, including early (10 to 13 years of age), middle (14 to 17 years of age), and late (18 to 20 years of age). During this time, child will go through many changes in his physical, psychological (mental and emotional), and social growth.

Information

During adolescence, children develop the ability to:

- Comprehend abstract content, such as higher mathematic concepts, and develop moral philosophies, including rights and privileges
- Question old values without a sense of dread or loss of identity
- Move gradually towards a more mature sense of identity and purpose
- Establish and maintain satisfying personal relationships by learning to share intimacy without inhibition or dread

Physical Development

Adolescence is characterized by dramatic physical changes moving the individual from childhood into physical maturity. Early, prepubescent changes are noted with the appearance of secondary sexual characteristics.

Girls may begin to develop breast buds as early as 8 years old, with full breast development achieved anywhere from 12 to 18 years. Pubic hair growth — as well as armpit and leg hair — typically begins at about age 9 or 10, and reaches adult distribution patterns at about 13 to 14 years.

Menarche (the beginning of menstrual periods) typically occurs about 2 years after initial pubescent changes are noted. It may occur as early as 10 years, or as late as 15 years, with the average in the United States being about 12.5 years. A concurrent rapid growth in height occurs between the ages of about 9.5 and 14.5 years, peaking somewhere around 12 years.

Boys may begin to note scrotal and testicular enlargement as early as 9 years of age, followed closely by lengthening of the penis. Adult size and shape of the genitals is typically reached by age 16 to 17 years. Pubic hair growth — as well as armpit, leg, chest, and facial hair — begins in males about age 12, and reaches adult distribution patterns at about 15 to 16 years.

A concurrent rapid growth in height occurs between the ages of about 10.5 to 11 and 16 to 18, peaking around age 14. Puberty is not marked with a sudden incident in males, as it is with the onset of menstruation in females. The appearance of regular nocturnal emissions (wet dreams), which may occur about every 2 weeks with the build-up of seminal fluid, marks the onset of puberty in males. This typically occurs between the ages of 13 and 17 years, with the average at about 14.5 years. Voice change in the male typically occurs parallel to penile growth, and the occurrence of nocturnal emissions occurs with the peak of the height spurt.

Behaviour

The sudden and rapid physical changes that adolescents experience typically lend this period of development to be one of self-consciousness, sensitivity and concern over one's own body changes, and excruciating comparisons between oneself and peers.

Because physical changes may not occur in a smooth, regular schedule, adolescents may go through stages of awkwardness, both in terms of appearance and physical mobility and coordination. Unnecessary anxieties may arise if adolescent girls are not informed and prepared for the menarche (the onset of menstrual periods), or if adolescent males are not provided accurate information about nocturnal emissions.

During adolescence, it is appropriate for youngsters to begin to separate from their parents and establish an individual identity. In some cases, this may occur with minimal reaction on the part of all involved.

However, in some families, significant conflict may arise over the adolescent's acts or gestures of rebellion, and the parents' needs to maintain control and have the youth comply. As adolescents pull away from parents in a search for identity, the peer group takes on a special significance. It may become a safe haven, in which the adolescent can test new ideas and compare physical and psychological growth.

In early adolescence, the peer group usually consists of non-romantic friendships, often including "cliques," gangs, or clubs. Members of the peer group often attempt to behave alike, dress alike, have secret codes or rituals, and participate in the same activities. As the youth moves into mid-adolescence (14 to 16 years) and beyond, the peer group expands to include romantic friendships.

Mid-to-late adolescence is characterized by a need to establish sexual identity through becoming comfortable with one's own body and sexual feelings. Through romantic friendships, dating, and experimentation, adolescents learn to express and receive intimate or sexual advances in a comfortable manner that is consistent with internalized values.

Young people who do not have the opportunity for such experiences may demonstrate difficulty in establishing intimate relationships into adulthood. Adolescents typically demonstrate behaviors consistent with several myths of adolescence:

The first myth is that they are "on stage" with the attention of others constantly centered upon their appearance or actions. This preoccupation stems from the fact that adolescents spend so much time thinking about and looking at themselves, it is only natural to assume that everyone else is also thinking and looking at them as well. In reality, this doesn't occur because "everyone else" (usually peers) is too preoccupied with their own issues. This normal self-centeredness may appear (especially to adults) to border on paranoia, narcissism, or even hysteria. Another myth of adolescence is that of the indestructible self. This belief feeds into ideation of "it will never happen to me, only the other person". In this sense, "it" may represent becoming pregnant or incurring a sexually-transmitted disease after having unprotected intercourse, causing an car crash while driving under the influence of alcohol or drugs, developing oral cancer as a result of chewing tobacco, or any of the numerous adverse effects of a wide range of risk-taking behaviors.

Safety

Adolescent safety issues stem from increased strength and agility that may develop before optimal decision-making skills develop. A strong need for peer approval, coupled with the myths of adolescence, may entice a young person to attempt hazardous feats, or participate in a variety of risk-taking behaviors.

Appropriate motor vehicle safety should be emphasized, focusing upon the roles of driver/passenger/pedestrian, the influence of substance abuse, and the importance of using seat belts. Privileges associated with cars and recreational motor vehicles should depend upon the adolescent's ability to demonstrate an adequate knowledge base and safe use of such vehicles.

Adolescents pursuing recreational athletic activities should be taught to use adequate equipment, protective gear or clothing, safe facilities, proper rules of safe play, and rational approaches to activities requiring advanced skill levels.

Young people need to be acutely aware of the potential dangers — including sudden death — which may occur not only with regular substance abuse, but even experimental use of drugs and alcohol.

Adolescents who are allowed to use or have access to firearms need to learn proper use, safety, and legal issues associated with guns.

If adolescents appear to be isolated from peers, disinterested in school or social activities, or deteriorating in performance at school, work, or sports — psychological evaluation may be necessary.

Many adolescents are at increased risk for depression and potential suicide attempts, due to pressures and conflicts that may arise within families, school or social organizations, and intimate relationships.

Parenting Tips

Adolescents usually require privacy in which to contemplate changes taking place within their own bodies. Ideally, the youth should be allowed to have a bedroom. If this is not possible, some private space should be allotted. Teasing an adolescent child about physical changes is inappropriate, because it may cause self-consciousness and embarrassment.

Parents need to remember that the adolescent's interest in body changes and sexual topics is natural, normal development and does not necessarily indicate movement into sexual activity. Parents must take care not to label emerging instinct and behaviors as wrong, "sick", or immoral. Adolescents may experiment with or consider a wide range of sexual orientations or behaviors prior to feeling comfortable with their own sexual identity.

A re-emergence of the Oedipal complex (a child's attraction to the parent of the opposite sex) is common during adolescent years. Healthy parents deal with this by acknowledging the physical changes and attractiveness of the child — and taking pride in the youth's growth into maturity — without crossing appropriate parent-child relationship boundaries.

It is normal for the parent to find the adolescent attractive, particularly as the teen often looks very similar to appearance of the other (same-sex) parent at an earlier age. This attraction may cause the parent to feel awkward, but care should be taken by the parent not to create disconnection, which may potentially make the adolescent feel responsible. It is inappropriate for a parent's attraction to a child to be anything more than an attraction as a parent. Attraction that crosses the parent-child boundaries may lead to inappropriately intimate behaviour with the adolescent, which is known as incest.

The teenager's quest for independence is normal development and need not be looked upon by the parent as rejection or a loss of control. To be of most benefit to the growing adolescent, a parent needs to be a constant and consistent figure, available as a sounding board for the youth's ideas without dominating or overtaking the emerging, independent identity of the young person.

Despite adolescents constantly challenging authority figures, they need or want limit-setting, as it provides a safe boundary in which to grow and function. Limit-setting refers to predetermined and negotiated rules and regulations regarding behaviour.

In contrast, power struggles arise when authority is at stake or "being right" becomes the primary issue. These situations should be avoided, if possible. Ultimately, one of the parties (typically the teen) is overpowered, causing the youth to lose face, and activating feelings of embarrassment, inadequacy, resentment, and bitterness.

Parents should be prepared for and recognize that there are common conflicts that may develop while parenting adolescents. The experience may be influenced by unresolved issues from a parent's own childhood, as well as unresolved issues from the adolescent's earlier years. Parents can anticipate their authority to be repeatedly challenged, as children enter and move through their adolescent years. Maintaining open lines of communication and clear, yet negotiable, limits or boundaries may prove useful in minimizing major conflicts. Most parents report a sense of increased wisdom and self-growth as they rise to the challenges of parenting adolescents.

DILEMMAS FACING HEALTH PROMOTING HOSPITALS

Defining the nature and impact of health promotion activities in HPHs leads to one of the main problems for the HPH movement. Most of the detailed activity would be more appropriately defined within the context of Health Educating Hospitals. Much of the available literature describes disease management objectives and outcomes alongside a particular focus on the promotion of 'smoke-free' hospitals. It appears that the fundamental HPH objective for moving away from pockets of health programme activity, which are primarily based on disease management/ avoidance activities, are seldom realised. This is not surprising, however, and perhaps inevitable given that many European countries stress the lack of government-related policy support, lack of individual organizational management commitment and lack of resources set aside for health promotion in hospitals.

A further dilemma that HPH initiatives face relates to the level and degree of organizational change that occurs in hospitals. Many HPH institutions state that their health promotion activities consist of a collection of health promotion programmes that may or may not be related to each other. The need for hospitals to adopt health promotion activities as core values within the organization, rather than institutions serving as organizations that merely deliver a few *ad hoc* health promotion projects, has been stated previously.

In essence, HPH initiatives are less likely to succeed where they fail to implement 'whole' organizational and cultural health promotion reform that influences the role and function of all health professional employees. This said, single hospital health promotion projects can be used as a vehicle towards the broader aim of wider development within the organizational setting and contribute to the organization's capacity to take on new initiatives. This can only occur though where the hospital then links individual projects and views them as a spring-board for a concerted and organizational-wide reform programme.

The HPH movement works on the assumption that health promotion improvement is the most effective vehicle for organizational development (Quinn *et al.*, 2001). Others concur with these sentiments but specify that their effectiveness depends on the methods and strategies that are used. Many are now championing the use of Action Research (AR) activities as a particularly appropriate means of implementing and evaluating 'whole system' health-promoting organizational reform. AR is seen by many as a method that fulfils both the enabling and the empowering goals of health promotion, as well as the principles of participatory learning that underpin preventative health education approaches. This said, my colleagues and I have already expressed concerns that the health promotion community has yet to take up this mantle concertedly (Whitehead *et al.*, 2003).

In line with the principles of organizational change strategies, the WHO (WHO, 2003a) states that 'the HPH project facilitates change to promote Total Quality Management (TQM) of the hospital'. Significant barriers to organizational development under this auspice, however, continue to exist. This can be criticized for the fact that TQM in its most limiting form does not support the ethos of health promotion reform in that it is management-focused and hierarchical.

In another form, however, TQM may be considered appropriate to use in light of more recent change-management and participatory Project Management (PM) reforms. It depends on the management philosophy of individual organizations as to how effectively whole organizational reform can be implemented through the marrying of management-related and health promotion programmes. Johnson (Johnson, 2000) has already stated that there are very few examples of institutional health promotion programs to draw upon. Viewing health promotion as a driving device that helps prompt the need for effective organizational change is a useful start (Ashcroft, 1996).

Perhaps the main driver for HPH reform in Europe is the capacity for hospitals to affect and influence public health reform and therefore directly influence the health of their surrounding communities. Hospitals and their leaders are being held increasingly accountable for the health status of local populations (Olden, 2003). This represents the greatest challenge for the HPH movement and perhaps its biggest failure to date. A broader vision would see the development of not just what could be termed as HPHs, but institutions that could be classified as Public Health Hospitals. A Public Health Hospital is one that develops its staff to move away from increasing medicalized subspecialization to an increasing understanding of the wider health agenda (Wright *et al.*, 2002). It does this as part of a health-promoting capacity-building process that leads to an organization's overall structural development, as well as offering a support structure for wider community health promotion initiatives through collaboration with public health agencies.

Johnson and Baum (Johnson and Baum, 2001) state that until a hospital is truly a health promoting organization in its own right, it cannot broaden its approach to improve the health of the community that it serves. Hospital services that are developed with little consideration of the systems that concern themselves in estimating the health needs of the local and wider community will remain insular and somewhat limited in their influence and scope.

Vang (Vang, 1995) argues that hospitals need to equally divide their health promoting activity into two categories: those that are directly aimed at reforming the institution and those that are aimed at reforming the surrounding community. According to Pelikan*et al.*:A health-promoting hospital promotes patients' health by ... using episodes of acute illness or injury as windows of opportunity to promote health, for instance by providing or organizing rehabilitation, and empowering patients to ... make better use of primary health care services ... It networks with the relevant local services and associations to build alliances for continuous care and health promotion, thus becoming an agent for health development in the community.

Achieving any sort of public health/community agenda presents a tall order for most hospitals in Europe. Indeed it represents a formidable challenge given some of the sentiments and apparent divisions that exist. For instance, Wright *et al.* assert that:Traditionally, public health professionals have scorned hospitals as the antithesis of community health. Secondary care remains notably distant from public health practice and policy ... hospitals are often viewed as being too downstream to be relevant to public health.

Weil and Harmata (Weil and Harmata, 2002) suggest that because of their need to focus on fiscal management issues, too many hospitals have now set aside their mission to promote and protect the health of their surrounding communities. Similarly, Guilmette *et al.* (Guilmette *et al.*, 2001) state that hospital priorities of reducing in-patient stay periods and other functional outcomes means that health promotion issues do not receive the attention that they deserve. If signed-up HPH organizations struggle to influence the health promotion agenda of their surrounding communities, to what degree can non-HPH institutions be effective? This said, some argue that any health promotion activity has the potential to tip the balance in favour of wider reform. For instance, Johnson and Baum suggest that:... although hospitals are the high temples of sick care, the extensive resources that they command mean that even a small shift of focus has the potential to bring about an increase in resources dedicated to health promotion and, in time, health benefits to a community.

Despite the difficulty of the task, it is nevertheless one that must be undertaken if hospitals are to avoid existing in 'splendid isolation' from wider health policy or the health of the communities that they serve, and where any health promotion activity is 'more symbolic than authentic' (Wright *et al.*, 2002; Olden, 2003). Whitelaw *et al.* (Whitelaw *et al.*, 2001) outline their Health Promoting Health Service activity, which widens the role of the hospital setting to this effect. Perhaps another way of looking at the issues faced is not so much looking to re-structure whole organizations/institutions or beyond in terms of whole health services, but to break things down into more manageable reform. As a means of promoting HPH's restructuring, practitioners could focus on 'health-promoting wards'. Coakley (Coakley, 1998) suggests that focusing on health promotion in the ward setting could facilitate a public health role if wards acknowledge the 'peripheral' services that are often associated with them.

Encouragingly, some examples do exist where hospitals have looked to or have developed health promotion outreach programmes that describe a partnership between community and hospital, but these are still few and far between.

Uddin (Uddin, 2001) suggests that hospitals can be viewed as self-contained community health centres in their own right. McKee (McKee, 2000), however, disagrees and doubts the extent to which hospitals can influence and deliver major improvements in community-related health. Stout's (Stout, 1995) prediction that many hospitals would begin to build 'fitness centres' as an extension of community outreach services has not come to fruition. To some extent, it could be argued that 'drop-in/walk-in' health centres, where they are available, serve as a bridging facility between hospital and community.

Part of the HPH initiative, however, appears to hinder rather than assist this process. The WHO has set up a HPH standards committee as mentioned above. Most of the standards refer to the self-contained goals of topic-specific individual behaviour change programmes. Unfortunately, there is only implicit rather than explicit mention of public health or health policy-related standards.

Hungary, in its 2002 Annual Report, states that the 'heterogeneity of different regions/networks makes it difficult to create universal standards' (WHO, 2003a). In addition to this, in 1999 the WHO and 'The Network' organized a conference in Phuket (Thailand) from which the Phuket Declaration and the 'Towards Unity for Health—Partnerships among Stakeholders' initiatives evolved (WHO, 2003b). The overall aim here is 'to improve the relevance and performance of the health service delivery system to better meet peoples needs' (WHO, 2003b). While it is implicit that the stakeholders and sectors mentioned might include hospitals in the network, there is a strong community emphasis within the programme and none of the existing projects directly involve the hospital setting.

Bringing hospital-based health professionals on board with the HPH movement has proved to be both complex and difficult. Blinkhorn (Blinkhorn, 2002) is critical of the fact that doctors, nurses and allied health professionals devote most of their time to clinical duties and, health promotion activities aside, often do not provide basic health education programmes. The WHO acknowledges that most hospital staff believe that health promotion is not part of their function (WHO, 2003a).

The medical establishment is notably the most difficult health professional area to target in terms of hospital-based health promotion reform. Johnson (Johnson, 2000) argues that it is very difficult for hospital clinicians who have been trained to think exclusively in terms of disease-based care to apply health promotion principles to their practice, while Blinkhorn (Blinkhorn, 2002) states that most medical funding agencies have actively resisted the opportunity to establish health promotion settings.

At the same time, it is difficult for health promotion, as a relatively young discipline dealing with highly complex interventions, to compete with the dominant culture of evidence-based medicine (Pelikan*et al.*, 2001). This said, there is a growing concomitant awareness of health promotion in hospitals, in line with the growing awareness of the limitations of acute medicine (Johnson, 2000). The challenge here is not just to try to provide a different type of health-related service provision, but to staff a service with professionals that are prepared to adopt a different health-related mindset (Wright *et al.*, 2002).

8

Hospital Management of Patients

Out-of-hospital cardiac arrest (OHCA) is a major cause of mortality and serious morbidity throughout many regions of the world. Although there have been major advances in resuscitation practice, the survival rate for patients with OHCA, with a few recent exceptions, has remained poor for over 30 years: most regions report a survival rate to hospital discharge of <10%. For many years, research has focused on optimising prehospital management, as described recently in this journal.

After return of spontaneous circulation (ROSC), the aim is to limit neurological disability by optimising cardiocerebral resuscitation. The optimum therapeutic strategy after ROSC for patients with OHCA remains unknown. Increasing evidence suggests that optimising post-resuscitation management using a standardised treatment protocol and a multidisciplinary strategy can significantly improve survival. With optimal post-resuscitation care, OHCA should no longer be perceived as a terminal event. In recent years, survival rates have started to improve significantly in some regions, probably because of multiple factors, which will be explored in this review. We will focus on the current status of post-resuscitation science and provide clinical guidance on the in-hospital management of patients with OHCA.

Pre-Hospital Care

The decision by the prehospital emergency medical service (EMS) provider on when and where to transfer patients with OHCA is key. The primary aim is to achieve ROSC, stabilise the patient rapidly at scene and then transfer. Patient transfer with continuing cardiopulmonary resuscitation (CPR) reduces the quality of chest compressions. However, with the new mechanical chest compression devices (eg, LUCAS (Jolife, Lund, Sweden) and AutoPulse (Zoll Circulation, Chelmsford,

Massachusetts, USA)) adequate chest compression quality can be maintained during transport. Patient destination is important. About 80% of OHCAs are cardiac in origin and likely to benefit from admission to a centre with acute coronary care facilities, including immediate access to percutaneous coronary intervention (PCI). Selected patients with a high suspicion of coronary obstructive disease, for whom ROSC is not achieved at scene, may benefit from early transport for coronary intervention while CPR is continued and this is an area of continuing research.

Early Hospital Care

The primary aim of post-ROSC care is to optimise cardiocerebral recovery. In-hospital aims include maintaining cardiac output and cerebral perfusion, optimising systemic haemodynamics and minimising ischaemia-reperfusion injury. The importance of optimal post-resuscitation care is highlighted in the recent 2010 International Liaison Committee on Resuscitation consensus on CPR science with treatment recommendations and European Resuscitation Council (ERC) guidelines.

Immediate Cardiac Management and Coronary Angiography

The commonest cause of ventricular fibrillation or ventricular tachycardia cardiac arrest is cardiovascular disease, especially myocardial ischaemia. In a study of 714 all-rhythm patients with OHCA referred to a tertiary centre in Paris, 435 (61%) had no obvious extracardiac cause and underwent coronary angiography—304 (70%) had at least one significant coronary lesion. However, it remains unclear whether the lesion was responsible for the arrest and whether patients after ROSC really benefit from immediate angiography and revascularisation. Patients with cardiac arrest have been excluded from most acute myocardial infarction trials, which has created a 'knowledge gap' for these patients. While non-cardiac arrest patients with ST-elevation infarctions clearly benefit from immediate angiography/PCI, we lack data for patients after cardiac arrest.

There is no consensus and clinical practice is variable among medical centres and cardiologists. An ECG should be recorded as soon as possible after ROSC to assess ST elevation or (new) left bundle branch block. The rationale for urgent angiography is that early revascularisation may minimise myocardial necrosis, which will increase cardiac output, reduce the likelihood of arrhythmias and increase cerebral blood flow. Several non-randomised observational studies have demonstrated survival benefit from early angiography after OHCA compared with no or delayed angiography/coronary intervention. However, studies have also highlighted an increased complication risk if early angiography is performed in these patients.

Angiography is often delayed until the neurological status of the patient can be determined accurately. A common perception among cardiologists is that patients with OHCA have a poor survival rate and often remain neurologically impaired—recent data showing favourable outcomes in these patients should change this view. Cardiologists and hospitals in the USA and some European countries, such as the UK, are being publicly scored according to their PCI outcomes and deaths from OHCA will adversely affect the overall rating of the hospital and the provider. This is problematic; the neurological status is difficult to assess reliably during the first few days after OHCA, especially in those undergoing hypothermia treatment.

Overall, it remains unknown which patients will benefit from early angiography/PCI after resuscitation from cardiac arrest. Guidelines advocate early angiography for patients with ST elevation on a post-resuscitation 12-lead ECG. However, the ECG has poor accuracy in this setting. The absence of ST elevation does not exclude the presence of critical coronary stenosis. In a recent study, the negative predictive value for a critical lesion was only about 42%, while 58% still had a critical lesion despite the absence of ST elevation. In approximately 50% of patients without ST elevation after arrest, a significant lesion was found and stented; however, evidence to support this strategy is lacking.

Unless there is a thrombotic occlusion, angiography is an insufficient method to detect vulnerable coronary lesions. Despite this lack of evidence, we strongly advocate that all patients with ROSC should undergo early coronary angiography if there is no obvious non-cardiac cause of the cardiac arrest, regardless of the initial post-ROSC ECG since the predictive value of the post-ROSC ECG is low. Early information about the coronary circulation can guide in-hospital management beyond a coronary intervention and, in patients in cardiogenic shock, an intra-aortic balloon pump or other support devices can be implemented immediately to improve cardiac output. In our opinion, an early angiogram provides more benefit than harm, but this strategy would have significant resource implications, especially in cardiac centres.

Therapeutic Hypothermia

Mild therapeutic hypothermia (MTH) is the only post-ROSC intervention shown to improve survival from OHCA in humans. Two randomised clinical trials (the Hypothermia After Cardiac Arrest (HACA) trial from Europe and a smaller trial from Australia) have demonstrated the efficacy of this intervention. The protective effects of MTH are largely unknown but are thought to include a reduction of ischaemia-reperfusion injury and limitation of oxidative stress. During cardiac arrest, brain tissue becomes ischaemic. After ROSC, rapid re-oxygenation leads to oxygen free-radical production, which can lead to secondary cell death. MTH has a pleiotropic neuroprotective effect. It slows down cellular metabolism, altering biochemical and signalling pathways, and reduces oxygen demand. Comatose (defined in the HACA trial as lack of response to verbal commands) adult patients with ROSC after out-of-hospital ventricular fibrillation cardiac arrest should be cooled to 32–34°C for at least 12–24 h. MTH can also be considered after OHCA with non-shockable initial rhythms such as pulseless electric activity or asystole but the benefit for these patients is less clear.

Many questions surrounding MTH remain unanswered. The timing of initiation and the optimal duration of cooling are unclear. Should MTH be started before admission to hospital or is it sufficient to start this treatment in hospital? Some experimental studies suggest that early cooling improves outcome; however, a clinical randomised trial failed to show superiority for prehospital cooling versus in-hospital initiated cooling. The timeframe during which MTH can be started is unknown. The length of time MTH should be maintained is also uncertain. In the Australian trial, patients were cooled for 12 h, while in the HACA trial they were cooled for 24 h. A longer duration might be better but could be logistically challenging.

The optimal cooling method is not yet clear. External cooling methods include cold pads and cooling caps, while internal cooling methods include cold intravenous saline or intravascular cooling catheters. Recently, intranasal evaporative cooling has been shown to produce effective prehospital cooling. However, 30 ml/kg of intravenous 4°C saline or Hartmann's solution is the simplest and most cost-effective method for the prehospital setting. The target core temperature is 33±1°C. Intravascular devices are effective in inducing and maintaining this target temperature; however, there can be delays in inserting the intravascular catheter and this is more invasive than other techniques. Surface cooling, using cooling blankets and ice packs to the axilla, groin and neck, has also been advocated. These devices are simple, require less operator experience and are inexpensive, but initial cooling may be slower. One study has shown that both intravascular and surface cooling are equally effective for reaching and maintaining core temperatures, although another study showed better temperature control with an intravascular device. Whichever method is used, a feedback loop is advocated to ensure target temperature compliance and to prevent overcooling. Devices with feedback control also enable better control of rewarming (usually at 0.25°C/h).

Despite strong evidence and clear guideline recommendations, MTH is still underused in some regions of the world. In a recent trial of an impedance threshold device for OHCA in the USA and Canada, just 48% of the 2289 enrolled patients admitted to hospital were treated with therapeutic hypothermia. On the other hand, in the UK 86% of intensive care units (ICUs) had implemented hypothermia by 2009.Lack of resources and cost of MTH are commonly cited as barriers to implementation, despite relatively cheap options being available.

Sedation After Cardiac Arrest

All patients with OHCA receiving MTH will have been intubated (prehospital or in hospital) and use of sedation (opioids, anxiolytics and sedative-hypnotic drugs such as propofol) will prevent shivering, assist control of ventilation and blunt the stress-related surge of endogenous catecholamines. Occasional bolus doses of muscle relaxant may be required but should not be given by infusion unless continuous electroencephalographic monitoring is available, otherwise seizure activity may be missed.

Systemic and Cerebral Circulation

Hypotension is common among cardiac arrest survivors admitted to the ICU. The optimum post-resuscitation blood pressure has not been defined but must be high enough to maintain cerebral perfusion despite impaired cerebral autoregulation but not excessively high because this will increase myocardial work. The target mean arterial blood pressure will be higher than 65 mm Hg but the optimal value will depend on the patient's normal blood pressure and the value that achieves an adequate urine output.

Global myocardial dysfunction, which can be quantified with early and serial echocardiography, is common after cardiac arrest but typically recovers over 48–72 h. Treatment with an inotrope, such as dobutamine, or an intra-aortic balloon pump may be required. Monitoring of cardiac output may be helpful because the inflammatory response associated with post-cardiac arrest syndrome may result in significant vasodilatation, which may require treatment with a vasopressor such as norepinephrine.

Ventilation and Oxygenation

Pulmonary dysfunction is common after cardiac arrest. Problems include pulmonary oedema from left ventricular dysfunction, infective or physical lung injuries, pulmonary atelectasis or aspiration occurring during resuscitation. In a recent French study, of 641 patients admitted after OHCA 419 (65%) developed pneumonia within the first 3 days. Patients often develop regional ventilation–perfusion mismatch, contributing to decreased arterial oxygen content. Hyperventilation should be avoided as it decreases cerebral blood flow and cardiac output.

During the initial stages of reperfusion excessive tissue oxygen concentrations may compound neuronal damage by increasing the production of free radicals, which damage mitochondria. In an animal study, ventilation with the minimum fractional inspired oxygen (FiO_2) required to maintain adequate oxygen saturation of arterial blood (94–96%), compared with 100% oxygen, during the initial phases of resuscitation (controlled reoxygenation) optimised neurological outcome.

These animal data are supported by a clinical registry study that included more than 6000 patients: based on the first documented arterial blood gas sample, post-resuscitation hyperoxaemia was associated with worse outcome than both normoxaemia and hypoxaemia. However, another clinical registry study of over 12 000 patients that used the lowest arterial oxygen pressure (PaO_2) value and controlling for more potential confounders (such as sickness severity) did not show a convincing association between hyperoxaemia and mortality. Based on these conflicting data, unnecessary arterial hyperoxaemia should be avoided, particularly during the initial post-cardiac arrest period. The 2010 ERC guidelines recommend that once ROSC has been established and the oxygen saturation of arterial blood (SaO_2) can be monitored reliably (by pulse oximetry and/or arterial blood gas analysis), inspired oxygen is titrated to achieve a SaO_2 of 94–98%.

Metabolic Monitoring

OHCA results in multiorgan ischaemia. Since abnormalities in baseline blood glucose, electrolyte and arterial blood gas values are associated with poor survival and functional outcome after OHCA, monitoring and control of these physiological values are important. There is an association between high glucose values and worse outcome after OHCA; however, interventional studies that actively lowered glucose did not provide clear evidence that this improves clinical outcome, especially in cooled patients. In general, intensive glucose control has repeatedly been shown to increase the risk for severe hypoglycaemia, which is associated with worse outcomes. Thus, ERC guidelines recommend that in adults with sustained ROSC after cardiac arrest, blood glucose values >10 mmol/l (>180 mg/dl) should be treated, but hypoglycaemia must be avoided.

Prognostication and Long-Term Outlook

Most patients surviving to hospital discharge have a good long-term functional outcome, but these represent less than half of all those admitted after OHCA. Acute prediction of neurological outcome following OHCA has received increasing attention in recent years. Many intensivists are still heavily influenced by the 'Levy criteria', defined in the 1980s. This prediction algorithm used absent pupillary or corneal reflexes at any time point, or absent or extensor motor response at 72 h, to predict a poor neurological prognosis.

In 2006, after an evidence-based meta-analysis, the American Academy of Neurology published carefully assessed practice parameters on this subject. At 72 h, incomplete recovery of brainstem reflexes, myoclonus, extension posturing or absent motor response to pain, and bilaterally absent somatosensory cortical evoked potentials (N20) were described as being associated with a 0% false-positive rate for poor outcome (ie, lack of awakening). Furthermore, serum neuron-specific enolase and cerebral MRI were regarded as promising to help in identifying patients with little chance of neurological recovery. Importantly, these guidelines were based almost exclusively on data from the prehypothermia era.

Recent data on patients undergoing MTH show that indicators of poor outcome, such as absent motor responses or incomplete recovery of brainstem reflexes on day 3, peak neuron-specific enolase values exceeding the previously proposed cut-off point of 33 μg/l, and even electroclinical status epilepticus or absent N20 responses on somatosensory evoked potentials, no longer provide a 100% prediction of a hopeless prognosis if used alone. This may reflect a biasing of prognosticators by hypothermia and/or a residual effect of sedation. In summary, a growing body of evidence is questioning the automatic application of the 2006 American

Academy of Neurology guidelines in predicting outcome from OHCA, especially in patients undergoing MTH.

Furthermore, preliminary observations suggest that early electrophysiological or serological variables may help prognostication in patients with MTH; these studies, however, should be confirmed in larger cohorts. While awaiting further research in this field (which is urgently needed), it is important to assess post-anoxic patients using multimodal algorithms, which minimise potentially catastrophic false predictions of poor outcome.

The long-term treatment of patients after OHCA will depend on the cause of the cardiac arrest. Patients with underlying ischaemic heart disease should undergo urgent complete revascularisation and appropriate secondary prevention; those with reduced systolic left ventricular function and those at risk for recurrent events should be considered for implantable cardiac defibrillators.

MEDICAL AND HEALTH SERVICES MANAGERS

Significant Points: Rapid employment growth is projected; job opportunities will be especially good in offices of health practitioners, general medical and surgical hospitals, home health care services and outpatient care centres. Applicants with work experience in health care and strong business and management skills likely will have the best opportunities.

Earnings are high, but long work hours are common. A master's degree is the standard credential for most positions, although a bachelor's degree is adequate for some entry-level positions in smaller facilities and in health information management.

Nature of the Work: Health care is a business and, like every other business, it needs good management to keep it running smoothly. Medical and health services managers, also referred to as *health care executives* or *health care administrators*, plan, direct, coordinate and supervise the delivery of health care. Medical and health services managers include specialists and generalists. Specialists are in charge of specific clinical departments or services, while generalists manage or help manage an entire facility or system.

The structure and financing of health care are changing rapidly. Future medical and health services managers must be prepared to deal with evolving integrated health care delivery systems, technological innovations, an increasingly complex regulatory environment, restructuring of work and an increased focus on preventive care. They will be called on to improve efficiency in health care facilities and the quality of the health care provided. Increasingly, medical and health services managers will work in organizations in which they must optimize efficiency of a variety of related services—for example, those ranging from inpatient care to outpatient followup care.

Large facilities usually have several assistant administrators to aid the top administrator and to handle daily decisions. Assistant administrators may direct activities in clinical areas such as nursing, surgery, therapy, medical records, or health information. (Managers in non-health areas, such as administrative services, computer and information systems, finance and human resources, are not included in this statement.

In smaller facilities, top administrators handle more of the details of daily operations. For example, many nursing home administrators manage personnel, finances, facility operations and admissions and also have a larger role in resident care. Clinical managers have training or experience in a specific clinical area and, accordingly, have more specific responsibilities than do generalists. For example, directors of physical therapy are experienced physical therapists and most health information and medical record administrators have a bachelor's degree in health information or medical record administration. Clinical managers establish and implement policies, objectives and procedures for their departments; evaluate personnel and work; develop reports and budgets; and coordinate activities with other managers.

Health information managers are responsible for the maintenance and security of all patient records. Recent regulations enacted by the Federal Government require that all health care providers maintain electronic patient records and that these records be secure. As a result, health information managers must keep up with current computer and software technology and with legislative requirements and developments. In addition, as patient data become more frequently used for quality management and in medical research, health information managers ensure that databases are complete, accurate and available only to authorized personnel.

In group medical practices, managers work closely with physicians. Whereas an office manager might handle business affairs in small medical groups, leaving policy decisions to the physicians themselves, larger groups usually employ a full-time administrator to help formulate business strategies and coordinate day-to-day business.

A small group of 10 to 15 physicians might employ 1 administrator to oversee personnel matters, billing and collection, budgeting, planning, equipment outlays and patient flow. A large practice of 40 to 50 physicians might have a chief administrator and several assistants, each responsible for different areas.

Medical and health services managers in managed care settings perform functions similar to those of their counterparts in large group practices, except that they could have larger staffs to manage. In addition, they might do more community outreach and preventive care than do managers of a group practice. Some medical and health services managers oversee the activities of a number of facilities in health systems. Such systems might contain both inpatient and outpatient facilities and offer a wide range of patient services.

Working Conditions: Most medical and health services managers work long hours. Facilities such as nursing care facilities and hospitals operate around the clock and administrators and managers may be called at all hours to deal with problems. They also may travel to attend meetings or inspect satellite facilities.

Some managers work in comfortable, private offices; others share space with other managers or staff. They may spend considerable time walking, to consult with coworkers.

Training, Other Qualifications and Advancement: Medical and health services managers must be familiar with management principles and practices. A master's degree in health services administration, long-term care administration, health sciences, public health, public administration, or business administration is the standard credential for most generalist positions in this field. However, a bachelor's degree is adequate for some entry-level positions in smaller facilities, at the departmental level within health care organizations and in health information management. Physicians' offices and some other facilities may substitute on-the-job experience for formal education. Bachelor's, master's and doctoral degree programmes in health administration are offered by colleges; universities, and schools of public health, medicine, allied health, public administration and business administration. In 2005, 70 schools had accredited programmes leading to the master's degree in health services administration, according to the Commission on Accreditation of Healthcare Management Education. For persons seeking to become heads of clinical departments, a degree in the appropriate field and work experience may be sufficient early in their career. However, a master's degree in health services administration or a related field might be required to advance. For example, nursing service administrators usually are chosen from among supervisory registered nurses with administrative abilities and graduate degrees in nursing or health services administration.

Health information managers require a bachelor's degree from an accredited programme and a Registered Health Information Administrator (RHIA) certification from the American Health Information Management Association. In 2005, there were 45 accredited bachelor's programmes in health information management according to the Commission on Accreditation for Health Informatics and Information Management Education.

Some graduate programmes seek students with undergraduate degrees in business or health administration; however, many graduate programmes prefer students with a liberal arts or health profession background. Candidates with previous work experience in health care also may have an advantage. Competition for entry into these programmes is keen and applicants need above-average grades to gain admission. Graduate programmes usually last between 2 and 3 years.

They may include up to 1 year of supervised administrative experience and coursework in areas such as hospital organization and management, marketing, accounting and budgeting, human resources administration, strategic planning, law and ethics, biostatistics or epidemiology, health economics and health information systems. Some programmes allow students to specialize in one type of facility—hospitals, nursing care facilities, mental health facilities, or medical groups. Other programmes encourage a generalist approach to health administration education.

New graduates with master's degrees in health services administration may start as department managers or as staff. The level of the starting position varies with the experience of the applicant and the size of the organization. Hospitals and other health facilities offer postgraduate residencies and fellowships, which usually are staff positions. Graduates from master's degree programmes also take jobs in large medical group practices, clinics, mental health facilities, nursing care corporations and consulting firms. Graduates with bachelor's degrees in health administration usually begin as administrative assistants or assistant department heads in larger hospitals. They also may begin as department heads or assistant administrators in small hospitals or nursing care facilities.

All States and the District of Columbia require nursing care facility administrators to have a bachelor's degree, pass a licensing examination, complete a State-approved training programme and pursue continuing education. Some States also require licenses for administrators in assisted living facilities. A license is not required in other areas of medical and health services management.

Medical and health services managers often are responsible for millions of dollars' worth of facilities and equipment and hundreds of employees. To make effective decisions, they need to be open to different opinions and good at analyzing contradictory information. They must understand finance and information systems and be able to interpret data. Motivating others to implement their decisions requires strong leadership abilities. Tact, diplomacy, flexibility and communication skills are essential because medical and health services managers spend most of their time interacting with others.

Medical and health services managers advance by moving into more responsible and higher paying positions, such as assistant or associate administrator, department head, or CEO, or by moving to larger facilities. Some experienced managers also may become consultants or professors of health care management.

Employment: Medical and health services managers held about 248,000 jobs in 2004. About 30 percent worked in private hospitals and another 16 percent worked in offices of physicians or in nursing care facilities. The remainder worked mostly in home health care services, Federal Government health care facilities, ambulatory facilities run by State and local governments, outpatient care centres, insurance carriers and community care facilities for the elderly.

Job Outlook: Employment of medical and health services managers is expected to grow faster than average for all occupations through 2014, as the health care industry continues to expand and diversify. Job opportunities will be especially good in offices of health practitioners, general medical and surgical hospitals, home health care services and outpatient care centres. Applicants with work experience in the health care field and strong business and management skills should have the best opportunities. Competition for jobs at the highest management levels will be keen because of the high pay and prestige.

Managers in all settings will be needed to improve quality and efficiency of health care while controlling costs, as insurance companies and Medicare demand higher levels of accountability. Managers also will be needed to computerize patient records and to ensure their security as required by law. Additional demand for managers will stem from the need to recruit workers and increase employee retention, to comply with changing regulations, to implement new technology and to help improve the health of their communities by emphasizing preventive care.

Hospitals will continue to employ the most medical and health services managers over the 2004-14 projection period. However, the number of new jobs created is expected to increase at a slower rate in hospitals than in many other industries because of the growing utilization of clinics and other outpatient care sites. Despite relatively slow employment growth, a large number of new jobs will be created because of the industry's large size. Medical and health services managers with experience in large facilities will enjoy the best job opportunities, as hospitals become larger and more complex. Employment will grow fastest in practitioners' offices and in home health care agencies. Many services previously provided in hospitals will continue to shift to these sectors, especially as medical technologies improve. Demand in medical group practice management will grow as medical group practices become larger and more complex. Managers with specialized experience in a particular field, such as reimbursement, should have good opportunities. Medical and health services managers also will be employed by health care management companies that provide management services to hospitals and other organizations, as well as to specific departments such as emergency, information management systems, managed care contract negotiations and physician recruiting.

Earnings: Median annual earnings of medical and health services managers were $67,430 in May 2004. The middle 50 percent earned between $52,530 and $88,210. The lowest 10 percent earned less than $41,450 and the highest 10 percent earned more than $117,990. Median annual earnings in the industries employing the largest numbers of medical and health services managers in May 2004 were as follows:

Federal Government	$87,200
General medical and surgical hospitals	71,280
Offices of physicians	61,320
Nursing care facilities	60,940
Home health care services	60,320

Earnings of medical and health services managers vary by type and size of the facility, as well as by level of responsibility.

For example, the Medical Group Management Association reported that, in 2004, median salaries for administrators were $72,875 in practices with 6 or fewer physicians, $95,766 in practices with 7 to 25 physicians and $132,955 in practices with 26 or more physicians.

According to a survey by *Modern Healthcare* magazine, median annual compensation in 2004 for hospital administrators of selected clinical departments was $76,800 in respiratory care, $81,100 in physical therapy, $87,700 in home health care, $88,800 in laboratory services, $90,200 in long-term care, $93,500 in medical imaging/diagnostic radiology, $94,400 in rehabilitation services, $95,200 in cancer treatment facilities, $96,200 in cardiology, $102,800 in nursing services and $113,200 in pharmacies.

Salaries also varied according to size of facility and geographic region. According to a survey by the Professional Association of Health Care Office Management, total 2004 median compensation for office managers in speciality physicians' practices was $72,047 in gastroenterology, $66,946 in dermatology, $66,207 in cardiology, $64,543 in ophthalmology, $63,801 in obstetrics and gynecology, $62,545 in orthopedics, $58,595 in pediatrics, $52,211 in internal medicine, $50,924 in psychiatry and $50,049 in family practice.

INPATIENT REHABILITATION FACILITY MEDICAL NECESSITY CRITERIA

In order for IRF care to be considered reasonable and necessary, the documentation in the patient's IRF medical record must demonstrate a reasonable expectation that the following criteria were met at the time of admission to the IRF:

- The patient must require the active and ongoing therapeutic intervention of multiple therapy disciplines (physical therapy, occupational therapy, speech-language pathology, or prosthetics/orthotics), one of which must be physical or occupational therapy.
- The patient must generally require an intensive rehabilitation therapy programme. Under current industry standards, this intensive rehabilitation therapy programme generally consists of at least 3 hours of therapy per day at least 5 days per week. In certain well-documented cases, this intensive rehabilitation therapy programme might instead consist of at least 15 hours of intensive

rehabilitation therapy within a 7 consecutive day period, beginning with the date of admission to the IRF.

- The patient must reasonably be expected to actively participate in, and benefit significantly from, the intensive rehabilitation therapy programme at the time of admission to the IRF. The patient can only be expected to benefit significantly from the intensive rehabilitation therapy programme if the patient's condition and functional status are such that the patient can reasonably be expected to make measurable improvement (that will be of practical value to improve the patient's functional capacity or adaptation to impairments) as a result of the rehabilitation treatment and if such improvement can be expected to be made within a prescribed period of time.
- The patient must require physician supervision by a rehabilitation physician, defined as a licensed physician with specialized training and experience in inpatient rehabilitation. The requirement for medical supervision means that the rehabilitation physician must conduct face-to-face visits with the patient at least 3 days per week throughout the patient's stay in the IRF to assess the patient both medically and functionally, as well as to modify the course of treatment as needed to maximize the patient's capacity to benefit from the rehabilitation process.
- The patient must require an intensive and coordinated interdisciplinary approach to providing rehabilitation.

Multiple Therapy Disciplines

A primary distinction between the IRF environment and other rehabilitation settings is the interdisciplinary approach to providing rehabilitation therapy services in an IRF. Patients requiring only one discipline of therapy would not need this interdisciplinary approach to care. For this reason, the information in the patient's IRF medical record must document a reasonable expectation that, at the time of admission to the IRF, the patient required the active and ongoing therapeutic intervention of multiple therapy disciplines (physical therapy, occupational therapy, speech-language pathology, or prosthetics/orthotics), one of which must be physical or occupational therapy.

Intensive Level of Rehabilitation Services

A primary distinction between the IRF environment and other

rehabilitation settings is the intensity of rehabilitation therapy services provided in an IRF. For this reason, the information in the patient's IRF medical record must document a reasonable expectation that at the time of admission to the IRF the patient generally required the intensive rehabilitation therapy services that are uniquely provided in IRFs.

Although the intensity of rehabilitation services can be reflected in various ways, the generally-accepted standard by which the intensity of these services is typically demonstrated in IRFs is by the provision of intensive therapies at least 3 hours per day at least 5 days per week.

However, this is not the only way that such intensity of services can be demonstrated (that is, CMS does not intend for this measure to be used as a "rule of thumb" for determining whether a particular IRF claim is reasonable and necessary).

The intensity of therapy services provided in IRFs could also be demonstrated by the provision of 15 hours of therapy per week (that is, in a 7-consecutive day period starting from the date of admission). For example, if a hypothetical IRF patient was admitted to an IRF for a hip fracture, but was also undergoing chemotherapy for an unrelated issue, the patient might not be able to tolerate therapy on a predictable basis due to the chemotherapy.

Thus, this hypothetical patient might be more effectively served by the provision of 4 hours of therapy 3 days per week and 1 ½ hours of therapy on 2 (or more) other days per week in order to accommodate his or her chemotherapy schedule.

Thus, IRFs may also demonstrate a patient's need for intensive rehabilitation therapy services by showing that the patient required and could reasonably be expected to benefit from at least 15 hours of therapy per week (defined as a 7-consecutve day period starting from the date of admission), as long as the reasons for the patient's need for this programme of intensive rehabilitation are well-documented in the patient's IRF medical record and the overall amount of therapy can reasonably be expected to benefit the patient.

Many IRF patients will medically benefit from more than 3 hours of therapy per day or more than 15 hours of therapy per week, when all types of therapy are considered. However, the intensity of therapy provided must be reasonable and necessary under section 1862(a)(1)(A) of the Act and must never exceed the patient's level of need or tolerance, or compromise the patient's safety.

The required therapy treatments must begin within 36 hours from midnight of the day of admission to the IRF. Therapy evaluations constitute the beginning of the required therapy services.

As such, they are included in the total daily/weekly provision of therapies used to demonstrate the intensity of therapy services provided in an IRF. The standard of care for IRF patients is individualized (*i.e.*, one-on-one) therapy.

Group therapies serve as an adjunct to individual therapies. In those instances in which group therapy better meets the patient's needs on a limited basis, the situation/rationale that justifies group therapy should be specified in the patient's medical record at the IRF.

Brief Exceptions Policy

While patients requiring an IRF stay are expected to need and receive an intensive rehabilitation therapy programme, as described above, this may not be true for a limited number of days during a patient's IRF stay because patients' needs vary over time.

For example, if an unexpected clinical event occurs during the course of a patient's IRF stay that limits the patient's ability to participate in the intensive therapy programme for a brief period not to exceed 3 consecutive days (*e.g.*, extensive diagnostic tests off premises, prolonged intravenous infusion of chemotherapy or blood products, bed rest due to signs of deep vein thrombosis, exhaustion due to recent ambulance transportation, surgical procedure, etc.), the specific reasons for the break in the provision of therapy services must be documented in the patient's IRF medical record. If these reasons are appropriately documented in the patient's IRF medical record, such a break in service (of limited duration) will not affect the determination of the medical necessity of the IRF admission. Thus, Medicare contractors may approve brief exceptions to the intensity of therapy requirement in these particular cases if they determine that the initial expectation of the patient's active participation in intensive therapy during the IRF stay was based on a diligent preadmission screening, postadmission physician evaluation, and overall plan of care that were based on reasonable conclusions.

Ability to Actively Participate in Intensive Rehabilitation Therapy Programme

The information in the patient's IRF medical record must document a reasonable expectation that at the time of admission to the IRF the patient's condition is such that the patient can reasonably be expected to actively participate in, and significantly benefit.

Physician Supervision

A primary distinction between the IRF environment and other rehabilitation settings is the high level of physician supervision that accompanies the provision of intensive rehabilitation therapy services.

For this reason, the information in the patient's IRF medical record must document a reasonable expectation that at the time of admission to the IRF the patient's medical management and rehabilitation needs require an inpatient stay and close physician involvement.

Close physician involvement in the patient's care is demonstrated by documented face-to-face visits from a rehabilitation physician or other licensed treating physician with specialized training and experience in rehabilitation at least 3 days per week throughout the patient's IRF stay. The purpose of the face-to-face visits is to assess the patient both medically and functionally (with an emphasis on the important interactions between the patient's medical and functional goals and progress), as well as to modify the course of treatment as needed to maximize the patient's capacity to benefit from the rehabilitation process.

Other physician specialties may treat and visit the patient, as needed, more often than 3 days per week. However, the requirement for IRF physician supervision is intended to ensure that IRF patients receive more comprehensive assessments of their functional goals and progress, in light of their medical conditions, by a rehabilitation physician with the necessary training and experience to make these assessments at least 3 times per week. The required rehabilitation physician visits must be documented in the patient's medical record at the IRF.

INTERDISCIPLINARY TEAM APPROACH TO THE DELIVERY OF CARE

An IRF stay will only be considered reasonable and necessary if at the time of admission to the IRF the documentation in the patient's IRF medical record indicates a reasonable expectation that the complexity of the patient's nursing, medical management, and rehabilitation needs requires an inpatient stay and an interdisciplinary team approach to the delivery of rehabilitation care.

That is, the complexity of the patient's condition must be such that the rehabilitation goals indicated in the preadmission screening, the postadmission physician evaluation, and the overall plan of care can only be achieved through periodic team conferences—at least once a week—of an interdisciplinary team of medical professionals. Interdisciplinary services are those provided by a treatment team in which all of its members participate in a coordinated effort to benefit the patient and the patient's significant others and caregivers.

Interdisciplinary services, by definition, cannot be provided by only one discipline. Though individual members of the interdisciplinary team work within their own scopes of practice, each professional is also expected to coordinate his or her efforts with team members of other specialties, as well as with the patient and the patient's significant others and caregivers.

The purpose of the interdisciplinary team is to foster frequent, structured, and documented communication among disciplines to establish, prioritize, and achieve treatment goals. At a minimum, the interdisciplinary team must document participation by professionals from each of the following disciplines (each of whom must have current knowledge of the patient as documented in the medical record at the IRF):

- A rehabilitation physician with specialized training and experience in rehabilitation services;
- A registered nurse with specialized training or experience in rehabilitation;
- A social worker or a case manager (or both); and
- A licensed or certified therapist from each therapy discipline involved in treating the patient.

The interdisciplinary team must be led by a rehabilitation physician who is responsible for making the final decisions regarding the patient's treatment in the IRF. This physician must document concurrence with all decisions made by the interdisciplinary team at each meeting. The periodic team conferences—held a minimum of once per week—must focus on:

- Assessing the individual's progress towards the rehabilitation goals;
- Considering possible resolutions to any problems that could impede progress towards the goals;
- Reassessing the validity of the rehabilitation goals previously established; and
- Monitoring and revising the treatment plan, as needed.

A team conference may be formal or informal; however, a review by the various team members of each other's notes does not constitute a team conference. It is expected that all treating professionals from the required disciplines will be at every meeting or, in the infrequent case of an absence, be represented by another person of the same discipline who has current knowledge of the patient.

Documentation of each team conference must include the names and professional designations of the participants in the team conference. The occurrence of the team conferences and the decisions made during such conferences, such as those concerning discharge planning and the need for any adjustment in goals or in the prescribed treatment programme, must be recorded in the patient's medical record in the IRF.

The focus of the review of this requirement will be on the accuracy and quality of the information and decision-making, not on the internal processes used by the IRF in conducting the team conferences.

Definition of Measurable Improvement

A patient can only be expected to benefit significantly from an intensive rehabilitation therapy programme provided in an IRF, if the patient's IRF medical record indicates a reasonable expectation that a measurable, practical improvement in the patient's functional condition can be accomplished within a predetermined and reasonable period of time. In general, the goal of IRF treatment is to enable the patient's safe return to the home or community-based environment upon discharge from the IRF. The patient's IRF medical record is expected to indicate both the nature and degree of expected improvement and the expected length of time to achieve the improvement.

Since discharge planning is an integral part of any rehabilitation programme and must begin upon the patient's admission to the IRF, an extended period of time for discharge from the IRF would not be reasonable and necessary after established goals have been reached or the determination has been made that further progress is unlikely. For an IRF stay to be considered reasonable and necessary, the patient does not have to be expected to achieve complete independence in the domain of self-care.

However, to justify the need for a continued IRF stay, the documentation in the IRF medical record must demonstrate the patient's ongoing requirement for an intensive level of rehabilitation services and an inter-disciplinary team approach to care. Further, the IRF medical record must also demonstrate that the patient is making functional improvements that are ongoing and sustainable, as well as of practical value, measured against his/her condition at the start of treatment.

Since in most instances the goal of an IRF stay is to enable a patient's safe return to the home or community-based environment upon discharge, the patient's treatment goals and achievements during an IRF admission are expected to reflect significant and timely progress towards this end result. During most IRF stays, therefore, the emphasis of therapies would generally shift from traditional, patient-centered therapeutic services to patient/caregiver education, durable medical equipment training, and other similar therapies that prepare the patient for a safe discharge to the home or community-based environment.

INPATIENT REHABILITATION FACILITY (IRF) SERVICES

The inpatient rehabilitation facility (IRF) benefit is designed to provide intensive rehabilitation therapy in a resource intensive inpatient hospital environment for patients who, due to the complexity of their nursing, medical management, and rehabilitation needs, require and can reasonably be expected to benefit from an inpatient stay and an interdisciplinary team approach to the delivery of rehabilitation care.

The IRF benefit is not to be used as an alternative to completion of the full course of treatment in the referring hospital. A patient who has not yet completed the full course of treatment in the referring hospital is expected to remain in the referring hospital, with appropriate rehabilitative treatment provided, until such time as the patient has completed the full course of treatment.

Though medical management can be performed in an IRF, patients must be able to fully participate in and benefit from the intensive rehabilitation therapy programme provided in IRFs in order to be transferred to an IRF. IRF admissions for patients who are still completing their course of treatment in the referring hospital and who therefore are not able to participate in and benefit from the intensive rehabilitation therapy services provided in IRFs will not be considered reasonable and necessary.

Conversely, the IRF benefit is not appropriate for patients who have completed their full course of treatment in the referring hospital, but do not require intensive rehabilitation. Medicare benefits are available for such patients in a less-intensive setting. IRF care is only considered by

Medicare to be reasonable and necessary under 1862(a)(1)(A) of the Social Security Act if the patient meets all of the requirements outlined in 42 CFR §§412.622(a)(3), (4), and (5). This is true regardless of whether the patient is treated in the IRF for 1 or more of the 13 medical conditions listed in 42 CFR §412.23(b)(2)(ii) or not.

Medicare requires determinations of whether IRF stays are reasonable and necessary to be based on an assessment of each beneficiary's individual care needs. For detailed guidance on the required qualifications of a therapist, required skills of a therapist, and medically necessary and appropriately documented therapy services. The policies in those sections describe a standard of care that should be consistent throughout the therapy disciplines, regardless of the setting of care.

Documentation Requirements

Medicare contractors must consider the documentation contained in a patient's IRF medical record when determining whether an IRF admission was reasonable and necessary, specifically focusing on the preadmission screening, the post-admission physician evaluation, the overall plan of care, and the admission orders.

Required Preadmission Screening

A preadmission screening is an evaluation of the patient's condition and need for rehabilitation therapy and medical treatment that must be conducted by licensed or certified clinician(s) within the 48 hours immediately preceding the IRF admission.

A preadmission screening that includes all of the required elements, but that is conducted more than 48 hours immediately preceding the IRF admission, will be accepted as long as an update is conducted in person or by telephone to document the patient's medical and functional status within the 48 hours immediately preceding the IRF admission in the patient's medical record at the IRF.

The preadmission screening in the patient's IRF medical record serves as the primary documentation by the IRF clinical staff of the patient's status prior to admission and of the specific reasons that led the IRF clinical staff to conclude that the IRF admission would be reasonable and necessary. As such, IRFs must make this documentation detailed and comprehensive.

The preadmission screening documentation must indicate the patient's prior level of function (prior to the event or condition that led to the patient's need for intensive rehabilitation therapy), expected level of improvement, and the expected length of time necessary to achieve that level of improvement.

It must also include an evaluation of the patient's risk for clinical complications, the conditions that caused the need for rehabilitation, the treatments needed (*i.e.*, physical therapy, occupational therapy, speech-language pathology, or prosthetics/orthotics), expected frequency and duration of treatment in the IRF, anticipated discharge destination, any anticipated post-discharge treatments, and other information relevant to the care needs of the patient.

If the patient is being transferred from a referring hospital, the preadmission screening may be done in person or through a review of the patient's medical records from the referring hospital (either paper or electronic format), as long as those medical records contain the necessary assessments to make a reasonable determination. However, a preadmission screening conducted entirely by telephone will not be accepted without transmission of the patient's medical records from the referring hospital to the IRF and a review of those records by licensed or certified clinical staff in the IRF.

The IRF is responsible for developing a thorough preadmission screening process for patients admitted to the IRF from the home or community-based environment, which is expected to include all of the required elements described in this section. However, such admissions may not necessarily involve the use of medical records from a prior hospital stay in another inpatient hospital setting unless such records are pertinent to the individual patient's situation.

Individual elements of the preadmission screening may be evaluated by any clinician or group of clinicians designated by a rehabilitation physician, as long as the clinicians are licensed or certified and qualified to perform the evaluation within their scopes of practice and training. Although clinical personnel are required to evaluate the preadmission screening information, each IRF may determine its own processes for collecting and compiling the preadmission screening information.

The focus of the review of the preadmission screening information will be on its completeness, accuracy, and the extent to which it supports the appropriateness of the IRF admission decision, not on how the process is organized. The "rehabilitation physician" need not be a salaried employee of the IRF but must be a licensed physician with specialized training and experience in rehabilitation. For ease of exposition throughout this document, this physician will be referred to as a "rehabilitation physician". All findings of the preadmission screening must be conveyed to a rehabilitation physician prior to the IRF admission. In addition, the rehabilitation physician must document that he or she has reviewed and concurs with the findings and results of the preadmission screening prior to the IRF admission. All preadmission screening documentation (including documents transmitted from the referring hospital or other prior inpatient hospital stay, if applicable) must be retained in the patient's medical record at the IRF. "Trial" IRF admissions, during which patients were sometimes admitted to IRFs for 3 to 10 days to assess whether the patients would benefit significantly from treatment in the IRF or other settings, are no longer considered reasonable and necessary. Such determination must be made through a careful preadmission screening prior to the patient's admission to the IRF.

REQUIRED POST-ADMISSION PHYSICIAN EVALUATION

A post-admission physician evaluation of the patient must be performed by a rehabilitation physician. The purpose of the post-admission physician evaluation is to document the patient's status on admission to the IRF, compare it to that noted in the preadmission screening documentation, and begin development of the patient's expected course of treatment that will be completed with input from all of the interdisciplinary team members in the overall plan of care. The postadmission physician evaluation must identify any relevant changes that may have occurred since the preadmission screening and must include a documented history and physical exam, as well as a review of the patient's prior and current medical and functional conditions and comorbidities.

In order for the IRF stay to be considered reasonable and necessary, the post-admission physician evaluation must be completed within the first 24 hours of admission to the IRF and must support the medical necessity of the IRF admission. The post-admission physician evaluation documentation must be retained in the patient's medical record at the IRF.

What to do if there are differences between the preadmission screening and the postadmission physician evaluation (within the first 24 hours of admission to the IRF): In most cases, the clinical picture of the patient that emerges from the post-admission physician evaluation will closely resemble the information documented in the preadmission screening.

However, for a variety of reasons, the patient's condition at the time of admission may occasionally not match the description of the patient's condition on the preadmission screening. This could occur, for example, if the patient's condition changes after the preadmission screening is completed.

In these cases, it is important for a rehabilitation physician to note the discrepancy and to document any deviations from the preadmission screening as a result. For example, if the patient's preadmission screening indicated an expectation that the patient would actively participate in an intensive rehabilitation therapy programme on admission to the IRF, but the patient is only able to tolerate a less intensive therapy programme on the first day due to an increase in pain secondary to a long ambulance trip to the IRF, the IRF does not have to discharge the patient since the clinicians fully expect the patient to be able to participate in the intensive rehabilitation programme the next day.

Instead, the reason for the temporary change must be noted in the patient's medical record at the IRF. In addition, the preadmission screening and the post-admission physician evaluation could differ in rare cases when a patient's preadmission screening indicates that the patient is an appropriate candidate for IRF care but this turns out not to be the case, either, for example, due to a marked improvement in the patient's functional ability since the time of the preadmission screening or an inability to meet the demands of the IRF rehabilitation programme.

If this occurs, the IRF must immediately begin the process of discharging the patient to another setting of care. It might take a day or more for the IRF to find placement for the patient in another setting of care.

Medicare contractors will therefore allow the patient to continue to receive treatment in the IRF until placement in another setting can be found. However, in these particular cases, any IRF services provided after the 3rd day following the patient's admission to the IRF (considering the day of admission to be the 1st day) are not considered reasonable and necessary. In these particular cases, Medicare authorizes its contractors to permit the IRF claim to be paid at the appropriate case mix group (CMG) for IRF patient stays of 3 days or less.

Required Individualized Overall Plan of Care

Information from the preadmission screening and the post-admission physician evaluation, together with other information garnered from the assessments of all therapy disciplines involved in treating the patient and other pertinent clinicians, will be synthesized by a rehabilitation physician to support a documented overall plan of care, including an estimated length of stay.

The overall plan of care must detail the patient's medical prognosis and the anticipated interventions, functional outcomes, and discharge destination from the IRF stay, thereby supporting the medical necessity of the admission. The anticipated interventions detailed in the overall plan of care must include the expected intensity (meaning number of hours per day), frequency (meaning number of days per week), and duration (meaning the total number of days during the IRF stay) of physical, occupational, speech-language pathology, and prosthetic/orthotic therapies required by the patient during the IRF stay.

These expectations for the patient's course of treatment must be based on consideration of the patient's impairments, functional status, complicating conditions, and any other contributing factors.

Whereas the individual assessments of appropriate clinical staff will contribute to the information contained in the overall plan of care, it is the sole responsibility of a rehabilitation physician to integrate the information that is required in the overall plan of care and to document it in the patient's medical record at the IRF.

In the unlikely event that the patient's actual length of stay and/or the expected intensity, frequency, and duration of physical, occupational, speech-language pathology, and prosthetic/orthotic therapies in the IRF differ significantly from the expectations indicated in the overall plan of care, then the reasons for the discrepancies must be documented in detail in the patient's medical record at the IRF.

In order for the IRF admission to be considered reasonable and necessary, the overall plan of care must be completed within the first 4 days of the IRF admission; it must support the determination that the IRF admission is reasonable and necessary; and it must be retained in the patient's medical record at the IRF. While CMS believes that it may be good practice to conduct the first interdisciplinary team meeting within the first 4 days of admission to develop the overall individualized plan of care, CMS believes that there may be other ways of developing the overall individualized plan of care. Thus, IRFs may develop this required documentation using whatever internal processes they believe are most appropriate.

Required Admission Orders

At the time that each Medicare fee-for-service patient is admitted to an IRF, a physician must generate admission orders for the patient's care. These admission orders must be retained in the patient's medical record at the IRF.

Required Inpatient Rehabilitation Facility Patient Assessment Instrument (IRF-PAI)

Medicare now requires that the IRF patient assessment instrument (IRF-PAI) forms be included in the patient's medical record at the IRF (either in electronic or paper format). The information in the IRF-PAIs must correspond with all of the information provided in the patient's IRF medical record.

SERVICES RELATED TO AND REQUIRED AS A RESULT OF SERVICES

Medical and hospital services are sometimes required to treat a condition that arises as a result of services that are not covered because they are determined to be not reasonable and necessary or because they are excluded from coverage for other reasons.

Services "related to" non-covered services (*e.g.*, cosmetic surgery, non-covered organ transplants, non-covered artificial organ implants, etc.), including services related to follow-up care and complications of non-covered services which require treatment during a hospital stay in which the non-covered service was performed, are not covered services under Medicare.

Services "not related to" non-covered services are covered under Medicare. Following are examples of services "related to" and "not related to" non-covered services while the beneficiary is an inpatient:

- A beneficiary was hospitalized for a non-covered service and broke a leg while in the hospital. Services related to care of the broken leg during this stay is a clear example of "not related to" services and are covered under Medicare.
- A beneficiary was admitted to the hospital for covered services, but during the course of hospitalization became a candidate for a non-covered transplant or implant and actually received the transplant or implant during that hospital stay. When the original admission was entirely unrelated to the diagnosis that led to a recommendation

for a non-covered transplant or implant, the services related to the admitting condition would be covered.

- A beneficiary was admitted to the hospital for covered services related to a condition which ultimately led to identification of a need for transplant and receipt of a transplant during the same hospital stay. If, on the basis of the nature of the services and a comparison of the date they are received with the date on which the beneficiary is identified as a transplant candidate, the services could reasonably be attributed to preparation for the non-covered transplant, the services would be "related to" non-covered services and would also be non-covered.

Following is an example of services received subsequent to a non-covered inpatient stay:

- After a beneficiary has been discharged from the hospital stay in which the beneficiary received non-covered services, medical and hospital services required to treat a condition or complication that arises as a result of the prior non-covered services may be covered when they are reasonable and necessary in all other respects. Thus, coverage could be provided for subsequent inpatient stays or outpatient treatment ordinarily covered by Medicare, even if the need for treatment arose because of a previous non-covered procedure. Some examples of services that may be found to be covered under this policy are the reversal of intestinal bypass surgery for obesity, repair of complications from transsexual surgery or from cosmetic surgery, removal of a non-covered bladder stimulator, or treatment of any infection at the surgical site of a non-covered transplant that occurred following discharge from the hospital.

However, any subsequent services that could be expected to have been incorporated into a global fee are not covered. Thus, where a patient undergoes cosmetic surgery and the treatment regimen calls for a series of postoperative visits to the surgeon for evaluating the patient's progress, these visits are not covered.

RELIGIOUS NON-MEDICAL HEALTH CARE INSTITUTION (RNHCI) SERVICES

Section 1821 of the Social Security Act provides for coverage of services furnished in a Medicare qualified religious non-medical health care institution (RNHCI), when the beneficiary meets specific coverage conditions. The beneficiary must have a valid election for RNHCI services and would otherwise qualify for care in a conventional hospital or post hospital extended care facility that was not a religious non-medical health care institution.

The Medicare programme will only pay for non-medical health care services furnished in RNHCIs. The programme does not pay for supporting religious services or payment for the religious practitioner. The cost of religious items/services and the cost of using a religious practitioner is a personal financial responsibility and not covered by Medicare.

Beneficiary Eligibility for RNHCI Services

A beneficiary may elect to receive care in an RNHCI based on his or her own religious convictions or to revoke that election at any time if for any reason he or she decides to pursue medical care. Section 1821(a) of the Act requires that as a condition for Medicare coverage, the beneficiary must have a condition that would qualify under Medicare for inpatient hospital services or extended care services furnished in a hospital or skilled nursing facility that is not an RNHCI if it were not for their religious convictions. When a beneficiary has an effective election on file with CMS but does not have a condition that would qualify for Medicare inpatient hospital or posthospital extended care services if the beneficiary were an inpatient of a hospital or a resident of a SNF that is not an RNHCI, then services furnished in an RNHCI are not covered by Medicare. A Medicare claim for services that were furnished to that beneficiary would be treated as a claim for non-covered services.

If the beneficiary only needs assistance with activities of daily living, then the beneficiary's condition could not be considered as meeting the Medicare requirements. Prior to submitting a claim to Medicare it is the responsibility of the RNHCI's utilization review committee to determine that the beneficiary meets the Medicare requirements.

If no valid election is filed or the election has been revoked and no new election is in effect, the beneficiary does not have Medicare coverage for services furnished in an RNHCI. Consequently, a Medicare claim for services furnished to such a beneficiary would also be treated as a claim for non-covered services. In those cases where a beneficiary is admitted to an RNHCI with a valid election, the submission of prior claim for medical services to the Common Working File will revoke the election during the course of the RNHCI stay. If this is the first revocation, the beneficiary may make a new election without any disruption to the benefit. If this, however, is the second or subsequent revocation, the applicable waiting period applies and the remainder of the stay is not covered by Medicare.

Election of RNHCI Benefits

For an RNHCI to receive payment under the Medicare programme, the beneficiary must make a written election to receive benefits under §1821 of the Act. To elect religious non-medical health care services, the beneficiary or the beneficiary's legal representative must attest that the individual is conscientiously opposed to acceptance of non-excepted medical treatment, and the individual's acceptance of such treatment would be inconsistent with the individual's sincere religious beliefs.

Religious non-medical care or religious method of healing means health care furnished under established religious tenets that prohibit conventional or unconventional medical care for the treatment of a beneficiary, and the sole reliance on these religious tenets to fulfil a beneficiary's total health care needs. Medical care or treatment means health care furnished by or under the direction of a licensed physician that can involve diagnosing, treating, or preventing disease and other damage to the mind and body.

It may involve the use of pharmaceuticals, diet, exercise, surgical intervention, and technical procedures. The signed and notarized election must include a statement that the receipt of non-excepted medical services would constitute a revocation of the election and may limit further receipt of payment of religious non-medical health care services.

The election is effective on the date it is signed, and it remains in effect until revoked in writing or by the receipt and filing of a claim for non-excepted medical treatment. The completed election form must be filed with the specialty contractor, a copy retained by the RNHCI provider and a copy provided to the beneficiary.

The term is intended to identify the kinds of medical services that can be provided to a beneficiary with an election for RNHCI services without revoking the election. Examples of excepted medical care include, but are not limited to the following:

- A beneficiary that receives vaccinations required by a State or local jurisdiction. This is compliant behaviour to meet government requirements and not considered as voluntarily seeking medical care or services; or

- A beneficiary who is involved in an accident and receives medical attention at the accident scene, or in transport to the hospital, or at the hospital before being able to make their beliefs and wishes known; or
- A beneficiary who is unconscious and receives emergency care and is hospitalized before regaining consciousness or being able to locate his or her legal representative.

"Non-excepted" medical treatment is defined as medical care or treatment other than excepted medical treatment. The term is intended to define the kinds of medical services that, if received by a beneficiary who has previously elected RNHCI services, would revoke the individual's election of services. Examples of non-excepted medical care could include but are not limited to the following:

- A beneficiary receiving medical diagnosis and/or treatment for persistent headaches and/or chest pains.
- A beneficiary in an RNHCI who is transferring to a community hospital to have radiological studies and the reduction of a fracture.
- A beneficiary with intractable back pain receiving medical, surgical, or chiropractic services.
- A beneficiary who has requested a physician to prescribe a wheelchair or other durable medical equipment item.

Note that the terms 'excepted' and 'non-excepted' care represent mutually exclusive conditions under §1821 of the Social Security Act. Medicare contractors may use the examples above in making determinations of excepted and non-excepted care.

Bibliography

Aiken, L., Clarke, S. P., & Sloane, D. M.: *Hospital Staffing, Organization, and Quality of Care: Cross-national Findings*, International Journal for Quality in Health Care, 2002.

Bach, S.: *Health Sector Reform and Human Resource Management: Britain in Comparative Perspective*, The International Journal of Human Resource Management, 2000.

Baker, J. J. : *Cost Accounting for Healthcare Organizations: Utilizing Information and Technology for Effective Decision Making*. McGraw Hill, 1999.

Baker, R. W.: *Health Care Finance: Basic Tools for Nonfinancial Managers*. Aspen Publishers, Inc. 2000.

Beaver, K.: *Healthcare Information Systems, Second Edition (Best Practices)*. AUERBACH. 2002.

Berner, E. S.: *Clinical Decision Support Systems: Theory and Practice*. Springer-Verlag. 1998.

Berry, L. and K. Seltman. *Management Lessons from Mayo Clinic: Inside One of the World's Most Admired Service Organizations*. McGraw-Hill. 2008.

Bryson, McDowell: Concierge: *Key to Hospitality: A Training Manual*, New York, Wiley, 1992.

Buchbinder, S. B. and N. H. Shanks. *Introduction to Health Care Management*. Jones & Bartlett Learning. 2007.

Caldwell, C. and J. W. Juran. *The Handbook for Managing Change in Healthcare*. American Society for Quality, 1998. .

Clark, Mona: *Interpersonal Skills for Hospitality Managers*, London, Chapman Hill, 1995.

Cohen, F. and O. Dahl. *Lean Six Sigma for the Medical Practice*. Greenbranch Publishing. 2009.

Davidoff, Donald M.: *Customer Service in the Hospitality and Tourism Industry*, Englewood Cliffs, Prentice Hall, 1994.

Donald M.: *Customer Service in the Hospitality and Tourism Industry*, Englewood Cliffs, Prentice Hall, 1994.

Dubois C.: *Human Resources for Health Policies: A Critical Component in Health Policies,* Human Resources sfor Health, 2003.

Eberts, Marjorie: *Careers in Travel, Tourism, and Hospitality*, Lincolnwood, VGM Career Horizons, 1997.

Elio, C.: *The Hospitality Law Desk Reference*, Miami, Southern Beverage Journal, 1994.

Emery, William H.: *The Chef's Guide to Practical Restaurant Cookery*, New York, Van Nostrand Reinhold, 1988.

Force M.: *The Relationship between Effective Nurse Managers and Nursing Retention*, Journal of Nursing Administration, 2005.

Goldsmith, S. B. *Principles of Health Care Management: Foundations for a Changing Health Care System,* Jones & Bartlett Publishers. 2009.

Gould D.: *Locally Targeted Initiatives to Recruit and Retain Nurses in England,* Journal of Nursing Management, 2006.

Graban, M. *Lean Hospitals: Improving Quality, Patient Safety, and Employee Engagement*Productivity Press. 2011.

Hoffman, Edward: *Project Management Success Stories: Lessons of Project Leaders*, New York, John Wiley & Son, 2000.

Ireland, Lewis: *Quality Management for Projects and Programs*, Upper Darby, PMI, 1991.

Jimmerson, C. L. *Value Stream Mapping for Healthcare Made Easy*. Productivity Press. 2009.

Jitendra K. : *Contemporary Tourism and Hospitality Management*, Kanishka, Delhi, 2006.

Kassak K.: *Human Resources for Health Planning and Management in the Eastern Mediterranean Region: Facts, Gaps and Forward Thinking for Research and Policy*, Human Resources for Health, 2007.

Kotler, Philip : *Marketing Places*: *Attracting Investment, Industry & Tourism etc*, New York, free press, 1993.

Kotler, Philip: *Marketing for Hospitality and Tourism*: New Jersey, Prentice-Hall, 1998.

Kovener, R. R. *Chart of Accounts for Hospitals*. McGraw-Hill. 1999.

Lewis, Robert C.: *Cases in Hospitality Marketing and Management,* New York, John Wiley, 1997.

Lucas, Rosemary E.: *Managing Employee Relations in the Hotel and Catering Industry*, London, Cassell, 1995.

Lunguzi J, Wyss K.: *Scaling up the Stock of Health Workers: A Review International Centre for Human Resources in Nursing*, International Council of Nurses, Florence Nightingale International Foundation, 2009.

Mathis R, Jackson J.: *Healthcare Human Resource Management* Second edition, Thomson South-Western, 2008.

Mehta, N. H. and D. J. Maher. *Hospital Accounting Systems and Controls*. Prentice-Hall. 1977.

Merhi M, Jamal D, Dumit N, Mouro G.: *Assessment of Nurse Retention Challenges and Practices in Lebanese Hospitals: The Perspective of Nursing Directors*, Journal of Nursing Management, 2009.

Neumann, B. R. and K. E. Boles. *Management Accounting for Healthcare Organizations*. Bonus Books. 1998.

Nightingale, M. : *Tourism Occupations, Career Profile and Knowledge*, Annals of Tourism Research, 1981.

Ozcan, Y. A. *Quantitative Methods in Health Care Management: Techniques and Applications,* Jossey-Bass. 2009.

Pantelidis, I.S. : *Evaluating the Consumer in Hospitality*, Annual Research Conference: London, 2010.

Powers, Thomas F. : *Introduction to the Hospitality Healthcare,* New York, Wiley, 1995.

Quinn-Mills, D., & Walton, R. E.: *Managing Human Assets,* Free Press, New York, 1984.

Rosemary E.: *Managing Employee Relations in the Hotel and Catering Industry,* London, Cassell, 1995.

Sheldon, P. J. : *Professionalism in Tourism and Hospitality,* Annals of Tourism Research, 1989.

Shortell, S. M. and A. D. Kaluzny. *Health Care Management: Organization Design and Behavior, 5th edition.* Delmar Centage Learning. 2005.

Shortliffe, E. H. and L. M. Fagan. *Medical Informatics: Computer Applications in Health Care and Biomedicine (Health Informatics.).* Springer-Verlag. 2000.

Slinn, Judy A: *Tourism: Management of Facilities,* London, Pitman: M & E, 1993.

Story, P. *Dynamic Capacity Management for Healthcare: Advanced Methods and Tools for Optimization.* Productivity Press. 2010.

Thomas, F.: *Introduction to Management in the Hospitality Industry,* New York, Wiley, 1995.

Timothy R.: *Cases in Hospitality Healthcare: A Critical Incident Approach,* New York, Wiley, 1995.

Umbreit, T. : *The Role of Education in the Tourist Industry,* Salt Lake City, University of Utah, 1987.

Index

S

T

U

V

❑❑❑